CHEMICAL-FREE KIDS

How to Safeguard Your Child's Diet and Environment

ALLAN MAGAZINER, D.O.,
LINDA BONVIE, and ANTHONY ZOLEZZI

TWIN STREAMS
Kensington Publishing Corp.
http://www.kensingtonbooks.com

This book presents information based upon the research and personal experiences of the authors. It is not intended to be a substitute for a professional consultation with a physician or other health-care provider. Neither the publisher nor the authors can be held responsible for any adverse effects or consequences resulting from the use of any of the information in this book. They also cannot be held responsible for any errors or omissions in the book. If you have a condition that requires medical advice, the publisher and authors urge you to consult a competent health-care professional.

TWIN STREAMS BOOKS are published by

Kensington Publishing Corp.
850 Third Avenue
New York, NY 10022

All Kensington titles, imprints, and distributed lines are available at special quantity discounts for bulk purchases for sales promotions, premiums, fund-raising, educational, or institutional use.

Special book excerpts or customized printings can also be created to fit specific needs. For details, write or phone the office of the Kensington Special Sales Manager: Kensington Publishing Corp., 850 Third Avenue, New York, NY 10022. Attn. Special Sales Department. Phone: 1-800-221-2647.

Twin Streams and the TS logo Reg. U.S. Pat. & TM Off.

ISBN 0-7582-0369-1

First Trade Paperback Printing: August 2003
10 9 8 7 6 5 4 3 2 1

Printed in the United States of America

This book is dedicated to children everywhere with the hope that one day they will all have the opportunity to develop to their fullest potentials. Perhaps the time will come when no child's chance for a healthy future will be compromised by greed, apathy, or ignorance.

Contents

Acknowledgments

We would like to thank Lisa Zolezzi for her vision, support, and encouragement that was the initial impetus and inspiration for this book; Donna Gates for sharing her thoughts, recipes, and coconut water kefir with us; Jane Hersey for her advice and support; as well as the Feingold Association of the United States for allowing us to include some of their recipes in this book.

We are especially grateful to Bill Bonvie for his steadfast, tireless help, contributions, and guidance.

We also would like to thank the people that initially helped make this book possible: Bob Samuels, Dick Bogomolny, Suzanne DeBoever, Becky Rosetti, Eric Sanders, Marsha Friedman, and Mollie Katzen.

Foreword

Today's parents—especially the parents of children who are plagued with serious health challenges or learning problems, or who behave in ways that don't seem to make sense—need all the help they can get. Prospective parents need help, too, in preventing their as-yet-unborn children from falling victim to a variety of physical, mental, and emotional afflictions.

Why are so many American children now being diagnosed with such problems as asthma, attention-deficit/hyperactivity disorder (AD/HD), autism, mood swings and depression, sleep disturbances, behavioral disorders, learning disabilities, chronic ear infections, obesity, and diabetes? The approach most practitioners take in trying to address the root causes of these conditions is based on a few conventional assumptions that are just not supported by good science.

One such assumption is that children have always had these problems, but we simply have not been as aware of them as we are now—a theory that's hard to defend, given the alarming surge in health and behavioral anomalies. Another assumption is that some mysterious, inherent brain defect may be to blame—a speculation that doesn't take into account the many correctable external factors that may be affecting our kids' brains and nervous systems. Then there's an additional assumption—that if indeed the child has an abnormality of some type, the only way to treat it is with continued doses of powerful drugs that simply cover up the symptoms and may even cause additional harm.

What happens in such cases is that children who are actually suffering from allergies or sensitivities to various chemicals and toxic substances in their diets and surroundings may never have the real source of their problem identified. Those who have been damaged by exposure to heavy metals or pesticides, for instance, or who have a vitamin or mineral deficiency might not receive the kind of therapy they need or have the actual chemical culprits removed from their environment.

Practitioners with such deeper knowledge are out there, but unfortunately, they are still in a minority. Therefore, it falls on parents themselves to be aware of the whole picture, to try to understand why a child might be having problems, and to create the kind of regimen and environment that will prevent such problems from afflicting their children in the first place.

This book is a beacon designed to guide you past the many toxic pitfalls facing today's parents—a do-it-yourself manual based on the proposition that raising chemical-free kids is the best way of assuring they'll grow into healthy and well-adjusted adults.

—Jane Hersey, National Director of the Feingold Association of the United States and author of *Why Can't My Child Behave?* (Pear Tree Press, 1996)

Preface

Back in the proverbial "good old days" of a century or more ago, the chief concern facing parents was simply whether their kids would survive childhood. That's because it was expected that a sizable number of infants and children would succumb to various infections that today are considered little more than minor illnesses.

But if medical advances have succeeded in marginalizing most causes of infant and childhood mortality, much of what passes for "progress" has come to increasingly threaten our children in other, more devious ways. Today, the question is not so much whether our kids will manage to reach adulthood, but whether they'll grow up with healthy minds and bodies.

Will they be among the countless victims of our growing epidemic of allergies and asthma? Will they become hyperactive, dysfunctional, and unable to learn or, worse yet, join the fast-growing numbers of kids now considered autistic (an as-yet-unexplained phenomenon reflected by the results of a recent California study)? Will they become dependent on drugs, either illegal or prescribed to modify their behavior in the classroom? Will their bodies become overweight and obese, even as their brains are nutritionally starved? Will they be prime candidates for the cancers and cardiovascular problems that now result in so many premature deaths?

The answers to these questions will be determined largely by the everyday choices we make as parents and guardians—on what we feed our kids for breakfast or allow them to have as snacks, for instance, and on whether we opt to avoid exposing them to toxic pesticides in their diet and in the environment we create in our homes and yards. Beyond such personal choices, the answers depend on how effectively we intervene in the actions of others—by letting school officials know that we don't want our kids sitting in classrooms that have been sprayed with poisons (and providing information on viable alternatives) and by making a point of telling our family dentist that we don't want our kids' teeth filled with material that contains mercury, to cite but two examples.

Complaints about things ranging from chronic fatigue, headaches, and stomachaches to light-headedness and an inability to concentrate are quite apt to be symptoms of something out of whack in your kids' environment and may be harbingers of far more serious problems—unless you step in and put their lives on a safer and healthier course.

Doing so will also serve to instill in your kids an appreciation of the value of healthy living habits at the youngest possible age. That's especially crucial at a time when children are constantly bombarded with images and propaganda promoting the very types of behaviors that are almost guaranteed to adversely affect their health, vitality, and learning ability as they grow into adulthood.

This book evolved out of Anthony Zolezzi's mission to inform parents about toxic threats to their children's health, a mission he has pursued in numerous radio and television interviews. It represents the synthesis of his vision and ideas with Linda Bonvie's extensive research and writing (with the aid of her brother Bill) on many of the topics covered here, and with Dr. Allan Magaziner's firsthand experiences and expertise in working with chemically injured people of all ages and observing how a diet high in chemical additives while deficient in nutrients can diminish both the length and the quality of our lives.

This book is designed to serve both as an easy-to-use guide to assist busy parents in reducing their kids' exposure to harmful chemicals and as a source of background understanding of how such toxic threats to our well-being have been allowed to proliferate. On a practical level, rather than offering an "all or nothing" approach, it outlines changes you can make almost painlessly in your diet and lifestyle. Even if you incorporate just a few of the suggestions into your daily routine, your kids (and you yourself) will be far better off—and you'll be on the right path to making sure that your kids grow into healthy, strong, intelligent, and stable adults.

The point to keep in mind is that you do have choices in these matters—and you can choose to greatly reduce, if not entirely eliminate, your family's exposure to harmful chemicals. And since toxic exposures can have long-lasting effects on a child's development (starting inside the womb), including negative impacts on behavior and the ability to learn; can lead to life-threatening illnesses, such as cancer; and have caused many people to become severely sensitized to even the slightest whiff of anything synthetic, the stakes can be enormous. But so are the rewards for turning your family's immediate environment into a haven from toxic materials and for training your kids to enjoy the benefits of a relatively chemical-free lifestyle.

This book can help you to provide your kids with a healthier future—hopefully, one in which the only reasons to visit the doctor's office will be to obtain preventive advice and have wellness exams.

PART ONE

DETOXIFYING YOUR FAMILY'S DIET

Saying No to Fake and Toxic Foods

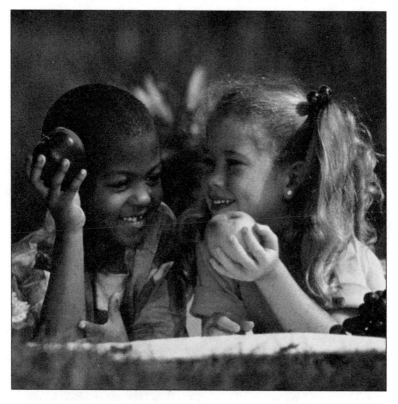

"Toxic exposures deserve special scrutiny because they are preventable causes of harm."
—*In Harm's Way: Toxic Threats to Child Development*
(Greater Boston Physicians for Social Responsibility, 2000)

WHAT YOU'LL FIND IN THIS CHAPTER

Kids need special protection. Infants and children are particularly vulnerable to the harmful effects of pesticides, which can include cancer and nerve damage. Typically, the younger a child is, the greater is his or her degree of susceptibility. Each exposure to a toxic chemical adds to a child's body burden, and since children can't detoxify as well as adults can, they need to be protected from pesticides and environmental poisons wherever possible.

Expectant mothers should avoid ingesting chemical additives. These substances, including pesticides and other toxic chemicals, can cross the placenta and affect the developing fetus. They're also apt to show up in the breast milk (which is generally considered nutritionally superior to infant formula).

Chemicals to be avoided in food whenever possible include:

- Pesticide residues
- MSG and hydrolyzed proteins, used as flavor enhancers
- Aspartame, the artificial sweetener marketed as NutraSweet and Equal
- Partially hydrogenated oils, found in baked goods and processed foods
- Bovine growth hormones, used to make cows produce more milk
- Artificial colors, artificial flavors, and preservatives

Doesn't the government safeguard the food we eat? While there are many dedicated people at both the Environmental Protection Agency (EPA) and the Food and Drug Administration (FDA), the way these watchdog agencies are set up makes it almost impossible for a food additive or pesticide to be restricted or banned once it has achieved an official "okay" to be on the market. Pesticides and food additives are supported and kept on the market by those who profit the most from their sale—the manufacturers. But you don't have to wait years for bureaucrats to take action against unsafe chemicals in your food—you can take action now to protect yourself and your family.

Our "protection" is at best a hit-and-miss proposition. Can the riskiest pesticides be regulated so that they can be used safely? That was the premise of a law passed in 1996 called the Food

Quality Protection Act (FQPA). It was to make pesticides "safer" for infants and children by finally acknowledging that kids are exposed to the same chemicals from numerous sources, that different chemicals can have similar effects on the body, and that some pesticides are so bad that kids need extra special protection from them. The EPA has until 2006 to complete the task, however, and some experts say its actions so far have watered down the law's intent.

Things You Can Do Now!

- Keep your kids' exposure to pesticides as low as possible. Daily doses add up, and the way kids play makes them more prone to ingesting pesticides than adults. For example, kids are more apt to absorb the pesticides from a treated lawn.
- Don't assume that pesticides are safe simply because the EPA allows them to be sold. Try to limit your family's dietary exposure to them by serving, whenever possible, organic foods, which are grown without pesticides.
- Read labels and shun such additives as aspartame, MSG, hydrolyzed proteins, artificial colors and flavors, and preservatives, as well as hydrogenated oils.
- Use organic dairy products. This is the only way to be certain you are avoiding bovine growth hormone.

"Where will she have her first French fry?" reads the poster hanging at McDonald's. The picture shows an infant, her perfect, tiny fingers resting in an adult's hand. So it's a given; not only will she absolutely, positively eat French fries, but her "first" will be a momentous occasion, ranking right up there with her first step and first day of school.

While French fries may not be the root of all nutritional evil, the message is clear: Your kids are part of the fast food culture from the day they are born, expected to go through life consuming whatever chemical-laden fare the industry decides to dish out to them. Nor are children the only targets of these commercial "body snatchers." Adults are also blitzed by a barrage of propaganda for health-destroying products, ranging from fat-and-additive-laden convenience foods to toxic chemicals that are touted as essential to saving your lawn from being defaced by alien dandelions.

We all know that something is wrong when asthma among children is reaching epidemic proportions, when hyperactivity and aggression have become commonplace in schools, when so many kids are being administered drugs to help them pay attention, when record numbers of children are being labeled as autistic, and when the National Cancer Institute attests to a 50 percent increase in childhood cancers of the brain and nervous system in the years from 1975 to 1998. It's becoming more and more apparent that the daily dose of toxins to which we're all exposed in our food, water, and environment is diminishing both the length and the quality of our lives. But children are those most at risk. How can we protect our kids, who are most susceptible not only to the effects of harmful additives and toxic chemicals, but also to the propaganda for the products that contain them?

BETTER CHOICES, HEALTHIER KIDS

It may seem like an impossible battle, taking on this ubiquitous commercial culture that's designed to sell us poisons for profit—until you remember that your home is your castle and no one's forcing you to open it to influences or substances that might be detrimental to the health and safety of the occupants. Armed with a little knowledge, you and you alone are empowered to refuse admittance to all the bad stuff that's out there trying to gain entrance to your living room, kitchen, and backyard. You can also take steps to protect your family from the various toxic and unhealthy influences on the outside. You don't have to feed your child that first McDonald's French fry, even with its reduced trans fat content, any more than you have to serve the chemical concoctions that are made to look like such fun foods on television.

In this book, you'll find out where many of the hazards lurk, how many better choices you have available, and how easy they can be to implement—beginning with the "ordinary" commodities that you bring home from the supermarket.

Why Kids Need an Extra Line of Defense

Kids eat differently than adults. They eat a more limited diet of "favorite" foods, and in relationship to their size, they actually eat and drink more than adults do. Because they are growing and developing, they are more susceptible to poisonous residues in foods, which accumulate in a child's body faster than they do in an adult's. And most importantly, their immune systems and brains are not fully developed. Although the brain may reach its full size by the age of sixteen, it's a long way from being finished.[1] The human brain is by far more complex than the most powerful computer and most vulnerable during its growth and "wiring" process.

What your kids eat for breakfast, lunch, dinner, and snacks may harbor some of the most insidious threats, both physical and mental, to their health and well-being. It could mean the difference between being asthmatic and being able to breathe freely, between being focused and being hyperactive, between having a calm, even-tempered disposition and having a tendency to fly off the handle, between landing in hot water and staying out of trouble, between failing and achieving in school, and between being healthy and being afflicted by illness in adulthood.

Once they've entered the world, it may seem to parents that children turn into "real people" relatively quickly. And in certain biological respects, that's true. For instance:

- A child's immune system undergoes its fastest development in the first six years.[2]
- Babies gain more weight during the first four to six months of life than at any other time.[3]

While development of the immune system, reproductive organs, and nervous system may begin before birth, it continues into childhood and adolescence[4]—and it can be seriously impeded by both exposure to harmful substances and a lack of proper nutrients. That's why it's essential that children be protected as much as possible from toxic agents in their diet and general environment (which isn't to say that their environment should be sterile, for as recent studies have shown, a relatively germ-free upbringing can make children more prone to asthma). But kids will be kids, and their habits can pose a challenge to a parent's most vigilant efforts.

When was the last time you crawled around the floor, saw something that caught your eye, picked it up, and put it in your mouth? Or routinely sucked your thumb after digging in the dirt? Or developed a fixation on grapes, squash, or bananas, flatly refusing to eat anything else? Probably not since you were a toddler. But it's just such everyday quirks and behaviors that help to increase a child's exposure to toxic pesticides.

Where kids are concerned, the potential for pesticide exposure is everywhere—at home, in day care, at school, on playgrounds, on carpeting (in the form of contaminants tracked in on shoes), and on food. Each exposure adds up in a kid's day, increasing his or her susceptibility to toxic effects. Philip Landrigan, M.D., chair of the National Academy of Sciences (NAS) committee that wrote the 1993 report *Pesticides in the Diets of Infants and Children*, noted that "it's children's aggregate exposure to many different pesticides that causes the trouble," adding, "of particular concern are exposures to pesticides in the family of organophosphates [one of which is chlorpyrifos, a recently restricted substance], because those chemicals were deliberately designed to be toxic to the nervous system. They have the potential to cause neurological [brain] injury to young children."[5]

The NAS report emphasizes that children are particularly susceptible to pesticides, given the poor protection they receive from federal regulations covering residues on food. The Environmental Protection Agency (EPA) itself has stated that the riskiest pesticides for kids need to be evaluated in combination, the same way they're eaten, not one at a time. Besides being subject to multisource, frequent exposures, a child's body can't detoxify poisons as well as an adult's. Rapidly developing bodies need special protection.

According to Dr. Landrigan, while there's no absolute cutoff time when a child becomes hardier or more resistant to poisons, "the general principle is the younger a child, the more vulnerable." This vulnerability starts before birth. "The growth of the brain is most rapid in the third trimester of pregnancy and in the first couple of years after birth," he says, adding, "some of these chemicals can cross the placenta from mother to baby."[6]

Harmful pesticide residues are contained not only in conventionally grown fruits and vegetables, but in such processed products as cookies, cereals, and even baby foods. While it may be easy to see the effects of acute pesticide poisoning, the subtle damage and illnesses that may develop years after chronic lower levels of exposure are difficult to pinpoint. The food industry and the companies that make and support the toxic chemicals that are sprayed, injected, and doused on our crops claim that small amounts of these poisons ingested along with our food pose no danger. But in reality, they don't really know.

Product Labels: When the Ingredients Belie the Hype

But pesticide residues aren't the only undesirable ingredients found in conventional foods. Potential threats to kids' health and development in the typical American diet are posed by a number of commonly used but potentially harmful additives, most of which are listed right on the labels—but which are all too easy to overlook, especially when the same labels contain misleading claims about the largely unnatural and adulterated products inside.

You have a right to expect the food you buy to be nutritious and wholesome, but the trend in conventional foods, especially in the "fast" and frozen varieties marketed for kids, has been steadily moving away from such values. In line with the "better living through chemicals" philosophy (to quote one corporate slogan) that took hold in the 1950s, the marketplace has been increasingly flooded by a stream of phony foods. Sprayed with poisons and laden with ingredients that have been modified, texturized, hydrolyzed, hydrogenated, and manufactured in laboratories, these products are often misrepresented as being "healthy."

You may think you're doing a good job of protecting your kids from bad dietary habits by steering them away from things like soda pop, chips, candy, and fast food burgers and fries, but these foods are only part of the problem. (And even if you make a point of excluding such items from your child's daily diet, they're often readily available right inside the schools themselves.) Perhaps even more of a nutritional threat are many of the processed foods you buy for breakfast, lunch, and dinner that are represented as "healthy" or "low-fat." In reality, such products are apt to be loaded with chemical additives—for example, artery-clogging trans fats and behavior-altering monosodium glutamate (MSG) in its various forms (both labeled and unlabeled). These products also tend to lack the nutrients necessary to promote proper growth and development. Yet given the demanding schedules of many of today's families and the fact that there's often so little time available to shop and prepare meals, it's easy to buy into such misinformation.

Misleading messages of this type, however, are being rejected by more and more parents these days—parents who have become increasingly aware that protecting their kids from becoming addicted to toxic, chemical-laden, nutritionally depleted food products is every bit as important as protecting them from becoming addicted to drugs or alcohol.

Identifying the Chemical Culprits in Your Kids' Food

"Let me warn you that you will be startled to discover how prevalent chemicals are in our daily diets when you begin looking for foods that don't contain them," wrote one of America's leading pediatricians, the late Dr. Robert S. Mendelsohn, back in 1984.[7] That continues to be the case today, but with a little extra effort, we can overcome the difficulties involved in finding foods that don't contain them. It is possible to substitute truly nutritious, natural food for the "convenient" chemical concoctions that we have long been persuaded to accept in lieu of the real thing.

The best part is that we don't have to totally alter our lifestyle

---

FOOD FANTASY
All Food Packaged for Kids Is Good for Kids

Sure, food packaged for kids has been designed to appeal to kids in terms of taste, gimmicks, and package design. But in terms of nutrition, the majority of such products couldn't be less kid-friendly. The amounts of sugar, sodium, and harmful additives they contain, coupled with the lack of those things that are essential to a child's physical and mental development, make them the dietary equivalent of Saturday morning cartoons.

For example, let's look at a popular frozen fried chicken "dinner" designed for kids. While it contains only two tiny "white meat wing drummettes," fifteen small pieces of French fries, about three tablespoons of corn, and a small pocket of chocolate pudding, it manages to have a whopping 850 milligrams of sodium, 440 calories, and 21 grams of fat—and that's the good part. The other ingredients include several partially hydrogenated oils, the artificial preservative butylated hydroxytoluene (BHT), disodium dihydrogen pyrophosphate (to promote color retention), modified food starch, cellulose gum, and seven artificial colors, as well as artificial flavors. In fact, you have to scan the label carefully to find words that you recognize as actual food substances. The package says, "Keep kids safe!" We think that an important part of keeping them safe is keeping them away from the kinds of "kids' foods" that are filled with chemical ingredients.

---

to introduce healthy change. If we're not quite ready to drastically alter our regimen—and let's face it, few of us are—our level of commitment to ridding our family's diet of harmful substances can be a gradual or a partial one. It can begin with something as simple as switching to organic cereal at breakfast or eliminating bread and cake that contain hydrogenated oil in favor of brands that don't. In time, one step can lead to another. It needn't be done all at once or ever be turned into a rigid ritual. The important thing is that we begin the process of phasing out disease-promoting chemical additives and replacing them with the kinds of things nature intended us to consume.

Let's begin by taking a brief look at some of the worst offenders (substances that we'll be discussing in greater detail later in this book). They include not only pesticides, but MSG and hydrolyzed proteins, aspartame, partially hydrogenated oils, bovine growth hormone, artificial colors, artificial flavors, and artificial preservatives.

Pesticides: Not Just Bad for Bugs

The widespread use of synthetic pesticides, growing steadily since the 1940s, has led us to complacently accept these chemicals as a normal part of the American landscape. How many times, for instance, have you seen kids and pets cavorting in grass amid little white warning flags or stopped to consider whether zapping a dandelion with herbicide was really necessary? Even school officials don't think twice about using these chemicals whenever they deem it necessary.[8] (The U.S. General Accounting Office reported at the beginning of 2000 that there was no comprehensive data on the amounts and kinds of pesticides being used in schools nor about the resulting illnesses in children.)

But things that by their very nature are designed to kill come with risks. And they don't always disappear after doing the job. Pesticides can remain in the air, food, and soil; contaminate water; and accumulate in plants, animals, and people. In fact, you don't have to make the choice between being overrun by insects or weeds and spraying your environment with toxic chemicals. Low toxicity and nontoxic alternatives do exist. (For more help with alternatives in your house and garden, see Chapter 5.)

If you found your child drinking from a bottle of insecticide or weed killer, your response would be predictable: You'd call the poison control center of your nearest hospital. Every day, however, 20 million children aged five and under consume an average of eight pesticides a day—along with the foods that are supposed to be "good" for them. These amounts may not produce immediate illness or symptoms, but their effects do tend to be cumulative, particularly in young, growing bodies. And they may well be reflected in health problems years later.

In Chapters 4 and 5, we'll talk more about the threat to your family's health posed by pesticide use at home and in school, but for now, we will stress that it is possible to immediately reduce your child's daily dose of pesticides. You don't have to move to a remote wilderness or grow all your own food to do so. Try incorporating the five tips that follow. If you can't do all five now, just pick one, but *start!*

Tips for Avoiding Pesticides

- Find nontoxic approaches to pest problems at home. (See Chapter 5.) Use chemical fixes only as a last resort, not as a first choice.
- Wash and peel conventionally grown vegetables and produce. (Veggies that don't get peeled should be washed very carefully.) It's also a good idea to remove and discard the outer leaves of some vegetables (such as lettuce).
- Rotate foods so that you're not eating the same things every day.
- Purchase organic foods, especially the ones you and your kids eat the most, whenever possible.
- If you have the space, start your own organic "Victory Garden." (See Chapter 7.)

MSG and Hydrolyzed Proteins: More Than a Headache

Monosodium glutamate, or MSG, gives the food to which it's added an advantage in terms of flavor the same way that steroids give an athlete the advantage of added physical strength. Not only are both unfair to the competition, but both can have harmful effects, especially when used over a period of time. But while you may be familiar with the MSG hangover commonly known as "Chinese restaurant syndrome," you may not be aware of the far more serious damage that continued consumption of MSG-laced foods can do to the brain and nervous system of a child or infant.

Children whose protective blood-brain barrier is not yet fully developed are especially susceptible to the effects of MSG. That's because MSG contains glutamic acid, a neurotransmitter, and the unregulated amounts to which kids may be exposed can have the effect of literally exciting brain cells to death. (Brain cells, remember, do not regenerate.) For this reason, MSG is often referred to as an "excitotoxin." The resulting damage will be discussed in greater depth in Chapter 2.

Now, you might think MSG is easy enough to avoid—just look for it on the label. Unfortunately, however, the component of MSG that triggers adverse reactions—processed free glutamic acid—is far more pervasive in processed food than first meets the eye. That's because it's also present in a variety of other additives found in products that range from snack foods to supposedly "healthy" frozen dinners—some, in fact, bearing labels that say "No MSG."

Perhaps the most common of these additives is the ingredient known as hydrolyzed protein (or variants like hydrolyzed soy protein). But there are others as well, such as caseinate (either sodium or calcium) and autolyzed yeast, which are contained in numerous products (take a look at the canned tuna in your kitchen cabinet, for instance). There are also others that are frequent sources, such as natural flavors, seasonings, and broths. Sometimes, you'll even find one or more of these in the same products that contain pure MSG—a double or triple whammy!

Tips for Avoiding MSG Reactions

- Check product labels for the presence of MSG, hydrolyzed proteins, and the various other forms of processed free glutamic acid.

- Inquire about ingredients when purchasing items from deli counters or eating in restaurants.
- Steer clear of foods with long lists of additives.
- Avoid foods containing hydrolyzed corn gluten and hydrolyzed wheat protein, both recently introduced ingredients that may contain "hidden" MSG.
- Avoid the newest artificial sweetener, neotame, which may affect MSG-sensitive people the same way aspartame does. (See "Aspartame: Sickeningly Sweet," below).

Aspartame: Sickeningly Sweet

Wishing to avoid the evils of sugar, many parents opt to feed their kids "sugar-free" or "diet" products in the mistaken belief that they represent a healthy alternative. But the artificial sweetener found in most of these items, a combination of chemicals known as aspartame (better known under the brand names "NutraSweet" and "Equal"), has proved to be anything but healthy for the many people who have reported suffering adverse reactions to it. This is evident in the thousands of complaints filed with the Food and Drug Administration (FDA) and consumer groups such as the Aspartame Consumer Safety Network. The symptoms described range from migraines to seizures to eye problems including blindness (possibly due to the fact that when aspartame breaks down, especially after it's heated, a toxic substance called methanol, or wood alcohol, that can damage the eyes and cause other problems as well, is released into the bloodstream).

But the potential harm from aspartame isn't limited to such complaints. Like MSG, aspartame contains a neurotransmitter, aspartic acid, that is also regarded as an excitotoxin, as well as phenylalanine, an amino acid that may alter brain chemistry by reducing levels of serotonin, a brain chemical that enhances one's feeling of well-being[9] (more in Chapter 2). And keep in mind that aspartame's effects tend to be most pronounced in what is probably its most common usage—as a sweetener in liquids such as diet soda.

Neotame, a recently introduced synthetic sweetener, is similar to but stronger than aspartame. Its approval by the FDA has drawn a good deal of criticism for having been based on inconclusive and less-than-adequate research, the results of which point to possible adverse effects that the agency ignored. (See more about neotame in Chapter 2.)

Tips for Avoiding Aspartame

- Be on the alert for the NutraSweet symbol on packaging and for aspartame in lists of ingredients. (Sometimes it's listed in very tiny letters and hard to notice.)
- Be particularly wary of products referred to as "light," "sugar-free," or "low-cal" (including certain so-called health foods).
- Avoid any product with a warning that it should not be used by anyone suffering from phenylketonuria (PKU), a relatively rare metabolic disorder. It's certain to contain aspartame, as you'll discover upon examining the ingredients.
- Avoid neotame, which was approved by the FDA in July 2002 for use in numerous foods and candies. Neotame has a chemical structure similar to that of aspartame, but with a potency thirty to sixty times greater.
- Avoid children's nutritional supplements and medicines containing aspartame; check product labels carefully.

Partially Hydrogenated Oils: Gumming Up the Works

They're not hard to find, being contained in the vast majority of cookies, baked goods, and cereals, not to mention a great many other processed foods (including supposedly "healthy" products, such as margarine). But the rap on hydrogenated oils (whether partially or fully hydrogenated) has finally been made public, and it isn't good. As the primary source of artery-clogging trans fatty acids in our diet, these chemically modified fats are now seen as a major contributor to heart disease, our nation's number-one killer. In fact, an expert at the FDA claims that removing trans fats from just a small percentage of bread, cakes, cookies, and crackers could prevent more than 17,000 heart attacks each year, many of them fatal.[10]

The purpose of hydrogenation—a chemical process that turns a liquid into a solid—is to increase a product's shelf life. But by doing so, manufacturers may also be decreasing your children's life expectancy, as well as your own. And while proposed new regulations would require the labeling of trans fats in food products, they won't make the foods containing them any safer. You don't have to wait for such labeling to protect your family, since you can safely assume that trans fats are present in anything with hydrogenated or partially hydrogenated oil among its ingredients. In fact, you don't have to check for them at all if you're eating certified organic products, in which they're strictly taboo.

Tips for Avoiding Trans Fats

- Look for hydrogenated and partially hydrogenated oils in all baked goods (such as cookies, bread, and pretzels).
- Look for hydrogenated and partially hydrogenated oils in processed foods (such as peanut butter and margarine).
- Use certified organic products whenever possible.
- Don't bake with margarine or solid shortening products.
- Use good oils (such as cold-pressed olive, coconut, or canola oil) in cooking and baking at home. (See Chapter 3.)

Bovine Growth Hormone: "Udderly" Unnatural (and Unhealthy)

Back in the 1950s, Hollywood liked to depict misguided (or "mad") scientists as tampering with nature, supposedly for the good of mankind, in ways that would produce catastrophic results—for instance, by injecting growth serum into laboratory animals, only to unleash a gigantic spider on the surrounding landscape. But what used to be science fiction has now become everyday scientific reality, and although we may not have succeeded in inadvertently creating monsters, we have managed to create unnatural conditions that may well result in some unforeseen and undesirable side effects.

A prime example is the use of bioengineered bovine growth hormone (BGH), now used to spur additional milk production throughout the nation's dairy industry (in a literal sense, "milking" the cows for more than their worth). Approved by the FDA in the early nineties after being referred to as a "manageable risk" (an evaluation that the Consumers Union found inappropriate in approving BGH, a veterinary drug used in food animals), BGH has since been at the center of a swirl of controversy.

For one thing, the hormone has a tendency to increase a cow's susceptibility to mastitis, an infection of the udders, which farmers are likely to treat with various antibiotics. This could possibly cause allergic reactions in some of the people consuming the milk from the treated animals, as well as contribute to the development of antibiotic-resistant strains of bacteria in our bodies.[11] But that may be just one of the potential problems associated with BGH, which a number of scientific experts have been warning may lead to a rise in the risk of certain cancers.

"Direct risks associated with the use of (BGH) in dairy cows appear to be related to the possible increase of IGF-I (another hormone) levels in milk," notes a report on its use by the European Union Scientific Committee on Veterinary Measures Relating to Public Health. "Risk characterization has pointed to an association between circulating IGF-I levels and an increased relative risk of breast and prostate cancer." The committee also noted that the possibilities of dietary IGF-I (insulin-like growth factor I) and related proteins present in BGH-treated cows leading to "gut-associated cancers" and gut-related problems in infants "need to be evaluated."[12]

But while it may be impossible to determine whether or not conventional dairy products come from BGH-treated cows, using certified organic products is a surefire way to keep BGH—and any associated risks—out of your family's diet.

Tip for Avoiding Bovine Growth Hormone

- Switch to organic dairy products, now available in many supermarkets as well as health food stores. This is the one and only way to be certain you're not consuming dairy products from BGH-treated cows.

Artificial Colors and Preservatives: Sources of Real Problems

While it may have more allure and last somewhat longer than unadulterated products, food laced with artificial colors and preservatives begins to seem a lot less appealing when you consider what it really contains and its possible effects on your family's health. Some artificial colors, for example, including Food, Drug, and Cosmetic (FD&C) Yellow Dye Number 6 and Blue Dye Number 2 (once derived from coal tar and now from petroleum), can provoke negative reactions; in addition, Blue Dye Number 2 has produced malignant tumors at the injection site when given to rats. The artificial preservative butylated hydroxytoluene (BHT), which is banned in England, can also cause adverse reactions, and studies have suggested that it (and chemical relatives butylated hydroxyanisole, known as BHA, and tertiary butylhydroquinone, called TBHQ) may be carcinogenic. Some of these effects will be discussed in greater detail in Chapter 2.

Tips for Avoiding Artificial Colors and Preservatives

- Avoid processed foods with artificial colors. (Did you really think the color of cherry gelatin comes from cherries?)
- Avoid the antioxidants BHA and BHT.
- Avoid propyl gallate, another antioxidant that may cause cancer.
- Steer clear of sodium nitrite, a meat preservative that interacts with other chemicals in food or the body to form powerful carcinogens called nitrosamines.
- Avoid sulfites, preservatives that can cause life-threatening reactions in sulfite-sensitive asthmatics.

Fluoride: Enough, Already!

For most people, the FDA-mandated warning currently found on toothpaste tubes about not swallowing the contents was the first inkling that fluoride, a chemical found in just about all commercial toothpaste brands, is a hazardous substance. For some, it may have been a rude awakening, since children (especially those less than two years old) are apt to swallow toothpaste involuntarily, and some adults do so deliberately to freshen their breath. Who would have suspected that something we've always been told was so beneficial might have a dark side? (While the warning found on fluoride-containing toothpaste packages says to "keep out of the reach of children under six years of age," the directions instruct kids as young as two to "brush teeth thoroughly . . . at least twice a day.")

As a parent, you're apt to accept as a "given" that fluoride is essential to keep your child from developing cavities. It's something you're still apt to hear repeated by most (although by no means all) dentists and health organizations, whose advice you might have little reason to doubt. You also probably take its safety for granted. (It's even being added to bottled water for children.) The trouble is that a growing number of scientists and health researchers, including staffers of the EPA, are now expressing serious doubts about this half-century-old conventional wisdom. And their concerns have been accentuated by some disturbing studies recently conducted by leading universities.

What we can say with certainty is that fluoride is a toxic substance (one often derived from industrial waste products) for which the EPA has set a maximum contaminant level in water (four parts per million). We also know that it can cause dental fluorosis, a permanent, unsightly discoloration of the teeth, and in larger amounts, a more serious condition called skeletal fluorosis, a potentially crippling bone condition. Whether current exposures can cause more extensive damage to bones and body organs (including cancer and nerve damage), as some scientists charge, is now being debated. (Studies, for instance, have found that "humans are being exposed to levels of fluoride we know alters behavior in rats," according to a report by Dr. Phyllis Mullenix, who has worked with both the Department of Psychiatry at Boston Children's Hospital and in neuropathology at Harvard Medical School.)[13] But whether or not you choose to believe those experts who urge that fluoride be avoided entirely, there's little reason to think that kids need any more than they're already getting from a variety of sources, such as soda, reconstituted juices, baby food, and practically every other processed product manufactured in a fluoridated community. To be on the safe side, in fact, it would be best to use nonfluoridated spring water (especially if your tap water is fluoridated) and one of several nonfluoridated varieties of toothpaste now available in health-food stores—which, you'll note, come without those mandatory "poison-control" warnings about not swallowing it.

Tips for Avoiding Excessive Fluoride Exposure

- Inquire whether your community tap water is fluoridated. If it is, purchase bottled water or install a water purification system that uses reverse osmosis.
- Since some bottled water has added fluoride, be sure to read the label before buying.
- Other products of which to be wary include kids' mouthwashes, which may contain a sizable amount of fluoride—and can increase the risk of poisoning because they come in "yummy flavors" and may be swallowed.
- Try to find toothpaste without added fluoride. (The best place to look is your health-food store.)
- If your kids use a fluoridated toothpaste or mouthwash, caution them not to swallow it. Better yet, supervise younger kids while brushing.
- Never allow very young children (who will involuntarily swallow substances) to use a fluoride toothpaste, and never use fluoride toothpaste as a gum rub on teething babies.

Genetically Engineered Foods:
Eating Like a Guinea Pig

Some people (particularly those whose livelihoods depend on big agriculture) will tell you that all the current fuss about genetically engineered foods is much ado about nothing, just talk about possible or theoretical harmful effects of which there are no actual proof. But that's just the critics' point—that such bioengineered products, in which genes from one organism are spliced into another to give it new characteristics, have been sneakily introduced into the marketplace without any real testing, and that therefore there is no actual understanding of their potential for adversely affecting either the environment or the people who consume them.

One such concern is the possibility of allergic reactions being triggered by exposure to substances in products in which they are not normally found. The allergic substances are in the products due to bioengineering, and consumers are totally unaware of their presence. As of this writing, for instance, several lawsuits, including a class-action suit, have been filed by individuals who claim they suffered adverse reactions after ingesting products containing StarLink corn, a genetically engineered strain not approved for human consumption due to just such a potential. While the StarLink strain wasn't intended to be used in this manner, it somehow managed to "slip in." At the same time that the StarLink-tainted products are the subject of a recall of extraordinary proportions (even though some of the involved companies insist that the corn is perfectly safe and should be approved as people food), other genetically modified (GM) items have already become well integrated into our food supply. And no one can say for sure what effects such "premature releases" might have on unwary consumers with varying degrees of food sensitivities.

This is good enough reason in itself to buy certified organic products whenever possible.

Tip for Avoiding Genetically Modified Organisms

- Buy products certified as organic or labeled as being free of genetically engineered or genetically modified organisms (GMOs).

WHY YOU CAN'T RELY ON THE GOVERNMENT REGULATORS

These days, a complaint one often hears (especially from business and industry representatives) is that government, by issuing excessive regulations, is acting like an overprotective parent. True, there's a vast federal regulatory apparatus in place that's theoretically supposed to be protecting us. But all too often, when it comes to the items that comprise our daily diet, the facts tell a different story. And the more familiar we are with them, the more it becomes evident that the job of keeping harmful substances out of our homes—and out of the food our kids consume—isn't one we can rely on anyone else to do. In reality, the job of being an "overprotective parent" (a label that those who have a stake in keeping us ignorant might tend to brand us with) is ours alone.

Where Have All the Watchdogs Gone?

It's a question that comes naturally: If so many things in food are harmful to us, and especially to our kids, how come the federal regulators—those watchdogs supposedly guarding our health at the FDA and the EPA—haven't taken whatever steps are necessary to eliminate such hazards from the food supply?

Some critics of those agencies would say it's because they have political and financial agendas and have become more interested in protecting corporate profits than consumers, with officials sometimes even being enticed to join the corporations they're obligated to regulate. While such criticism may not be completely unjustified, it's also unfair to the many dedicated individuals who give the job their best effort. A better answer might be that the manner in which these agencies are set up often makes effective regulation of all but the most blatant health hazards an unlikely proposition.

Take pesticides, for instance. While the EPA's job is to regulate their use and establish tolerances—that is, the legal limit allowed to remain on food—toxicity testing is a job that's been left up to the manufacturers to carry out, with results reported to the regulators. Now, under the provisions of the Food Quality Protection Act (FQPA) of 1996, many pesticides—nearly 450 of them formulated into thousands of products—are in the process of being reassessed, with an eye to decreasing the risk they pose to children. But that will take a tremendous amount of work, involving many products that have long been on the market. One such pesticide, chlorpyrifos, more commonly known as Dursban, was actually ordered removed from household products in the year 2000—a dramatic development, considering its many uses in homes and schools.

The problem, however, is one that has taken many years to develop, years in which poisons such as chlorpyrifos have come to be regarded as an indispensable part of life on the conventional farm. And even the most dedicated staffers at the EPA have only limited power and ability to deal with it.

The same holds true for the FDA, which is charged with regulating food additives. It, too, must rely on test-result data supplied by manufacturers. In addition, it is largely constrained by the manner in which it is obliged to operate—one that involves a list of "generally recognized as safe" foods established in 1958 and the following years, as opposed to others in the "food additives" category. Just how far the agency should go in setting safety standards for such products, however, is a source of much debate.

Then, too, there has evolved within the agency an emphasis on working with the representatives of large industries to arrive at cooperative forms of implementation—a far cry from what Dr. Harvey Washington Wiley, chief of the Department of Agriculture's Bureau of Chemistry, had in mind when he spurred Congress to pass the Pure Food and Drug Act nearly a century ago. Dr. Wiley, it should be noted, also studied the reactions of human volunteers—his "Poison Squad"—to determine the effects of various products on people, whereas today's FDA relies on animal testing and the opinions of scientific advisers. Even that system, however, isn't immune to outside influences, as was demonstrated in the early 1980s when aspartame was approved by the FDA commissioner at the time, Arthur Hull Hayes, a Reagan-era appointee who chose to ignore both unfavorable safety test results and the advice of the agency's own scientific experts.

Finally, there is the basic question of precisely who's in charge. As journalist Eric Schlosser notes in his book *Fast Food Nation* (Houghton Mifflin, 2001), there are currently no less than a dozen federal agencies, overseen by some twenty-eight congressional committees, with responsibility for food safety. Typical of the absurdities resulting from this situation, as Schlosser points out, is the fact that the FDA regulates the manufacture of frozen cheese pizza, unless it has pepperoni added, in which case it comes under the jurisdiction of the U.S. Department of Agriculture (USDA). Further compounding the gaps and confusion created by this patchwork-quilt approach to regulation is the dual responsibility of the USDA for both promoting and regulating agriculture at the same time.[14]

The regulatory watchdogs, in essence, are often simply unable to do the kind of thorough job of protecting us that we might assume they are doing. In addition to having too much responsibility and covering too wide an area, they're apt to be on short leashes—and may, at times, even be muzzled. That's why it's largely up to us to keep food-borne threats to the health and safety of our families from being allowed entry to our homes and our lives.

Food Fantasy
It Wouldn't Be for Sale If It Wasn't Safe to Eat

This popular misconception is one based on an erroneous idea of the role and the wisdom of the government regulators—the assumption that they know in all instances what's good for us and what isn't. Government agencies overlook many hazards to our health and well-being, often acting only when the evidence of harm becomes overwhelming. And keep in mind that safety testing is the responsibility of those who profit from the sale of a product.

The fact that so many items are regularly recalled should be enough to convince us of the need for vigilance. Products don't become "safe" simply by virtue of being sold in our neighborhood supermarket. It's up to us to monitor the safety of what our children eat, using both information and common sense.

We have witnessed many food preservatives, chemicals, additives, and medications being recalled after years of usage when enough adverse reactions were filed with the FDA. Also, most food chemicals have been tested only for toxicity or potential to cause cancer, but many kids experience hyperactivity, headaches, fatigue, or muscle aches and pains, which often are not addressed when these food components are tested.

The FQPA: "Protection" Built on a Faulty Promise

The EPA's reevaluation of chlorpyrifos is the most dramatic result so far of a new law unanimously passed by Congress in 1996—one designed to protect the most vulnerable segment of the American public from pesticide-related health risks that have previously been overlooked. Dubbed the "peace of mind guarantee" by former President Clinton, the Food Quality Protection Act (FQPA) is intended to establish "reasonable certainty that no harm will result to infants and children from aggregate (that is, multisource) exposure" to any particular pesticide. Under this law, the EPA must review all tolerances that were in effect up to the time of the law's passage—a total of 9,721. Some of the chemicals involved have been on the market for more than forty years.

To people concerned about their family's health, that may all sound very reassuring, holding out the promise that the conventional food they buy will have been thoroughly analyzed and declared relatively poison-free. Whether this much-ballyhooed legislation can even begin to live up to that covenant, however, is a different matter entirely, one that inspires little confidence among consumer advocates.

Passage of the FQPA was largely the result of a 1993 NAS report, *Pesticides in the Diets of Infants and Children*, which sounded the alarm about the extra risk these chemicals pose during the early stages of children's development. The law is one that supposedly obligates the EPA to establish more stringent standards for some of the most neurotoxic and widely applied pesticides. It also calls on the agency to reassess the cumulative risks of these chemicals. When pesticides have been studied for possible toxicity or adverse effects, they generally have been evaluated as single agents. The full effect of exposure to multiple pesticides is not well known, and their impacts on infants, toddlers, and children have never been studied.

What we do know is that pesticides can bioaccumulate in the fatty tissue of humans, concentrating in the organs containing the most fat—that is, the brain and the liver. Furthermore, every cell in our body is lined by a cell membrane that is composed of a fatty bilayer (membrane). Pesticides can therefore accumulate in every cell in the body and remain there for years.

The FQPA's key provision requires the EPA to apply an additional "tenfold margin of safety" whenever it lacks "reliable data" on prenatal and postnatal toxicity and on infant's and children's exposure to a particular chemical. It is the question of just what constitutes "reliable data," however, that some critics feel gives regulators room to wiggle out of the commitment. Dr. David Wallinga, former senior scientist with the Natural Resources Defense Council (NRDC), for instance, interpreted the phrase to mean

that the EPA must review and find adequate a whole list of perti-
nent data, ranging from toxicity findings (derived from in-utero
studies of test animals) to actual data on children's levels of exposure from all sources. At least, that's what he advised the EPA
back in 1998. But instead, the agency, according to Wallinga, "went
back and looked at the old testing requirements and decided they
were basically okay after all for purposes of complete and reliable
data. They argued that the tests they had all along provided that
information."

Also at issue was the timetable for implementing the new law.
Even if the review of all pesticides now registered was to go according to schedule (which, as of this writing, has not been the
case), the EPA has until 2006 to get the job done. Originally, a
third of the 875 active pesticide ingredients registered by the
EPA—those considered riskiest, including the organophosphates—were due to have been reviewed by mid-1999. (These ingredients are actually used in about 21,000 different products,[15]
and usually possess multiple registrations to fit the different commodities to which they can be legally applied.) When the EPA
failed to meet that deadline, noted Wallinga (who subsequently
went to work for the Institute of Agriculture and Trade Policy in
Minneapolis), the NRDC sued, finally coming to a settlement
agreement with the EPA to do the reassessment on a more timely
basis. In the meantime, the EPA did issue a "data call-in" (whereby
companies that have an interest in a particular chemical are asked
to submit more data on that pesticide's health effects) for about
140 pesticides "that were already known to be neurotoxic, because
they were designed that way." But progress was further stalled
after the "industry claimed they needed a brand new protocol"
(the set of instructions on how to perform a test), resulting in a
year of negotiations "just to agree on how to do it." As a result,
Wallinga maintains, there have been little, if any, new data gener-
ated outside of about nine studies already submitted to the
agency.

Some of these chemicals, Wallinga points out, "have been on

the market for over 40 years, yet we still can't get them tested to determine their effects on a child's brain. Even more shocking is that only two have been specifically tested for their effects on the immune system. And remember, asthma is an immune-mediated disease."[16]

Doubts about the process were reinforced in July 2002, when a five-member scientific advisory panel determined that the EPA had been premature in concluding that twenty-eight of thirty organophosphate pesticides are safe without adequately reviewing whether they are harmful when combined. The panel members contended that a threefold safety margin used by the agency, rather than the FQPA's tenfold factor, was not sufficient to assure adequate protection, and that the EPA had data on only six of the thirty pesticides when it made the decision. Upon learning of the panel's conclusion, a senior scientist for the Natural Resources Defense Council remarked, "This was so sloppy even the scientific advisory panel couldn't stomach it." (One of the two chemicals that the EPA declined to declare safe was dichlorvos, or DDVP, the substance used in the pest strips that are commonly found in many homes.)

Adam Goldberg, a policy analyst for the Consumers Union, concurs that the FQPA has so far largely failed to live up to the initial hype. "For most pesticides, they really don't have developmental neurotoxicity data," he maintains. "The EPA really hasn't done that in most cases. They should have done more—and they should have done it quicker."[17]

But perhaps it's unfair to place the entire responsibility on the EPA when the very promise of protection that the law provides may be a faulty one. "The whole intent of the FQPA was to come up with a risk-assessment formula that would permit [the riskiest] compounds to be used safely," says Dr. Landrigan. But he admits that the concept of the FQPA "moves in the direction of being an oxymoron. That's why a lot of parents are buying organic food," he adds.[18]

PROVIDING PRENATAL AND
POSTNATAL PROTECTION

In recent years, a lot of publicity has been given to a condition called "fetal alcohol syndrome," a mental and personality disorder suffered by children whose mothers became intoxicated during pregnancy. Less obvious, perhaps, is the damage that may be done to an unborn child by its mother having either exposed it to toxic substances in food or else failed to provide it with adequate nourishment while in the womb. Those nine months, after all, are the critical period during which cells are engaged in the complex task of organizing themselves into organs. In that endeavor, they need all the help they can get from the proper combinations of essential vitamins, minerals, proteins, and fats. By the same token, they need to be protected from having the job sabotaged by the intrusion of "cell-molesting" chemicals.

A growing number of mothers-to-be have come to realize that bringing up chemical-free, nutritionally advantaged children is a process that begins during prenatal development and have changed their own dietary habits accordingly. They're giving up chemically flavored and preserved, pesticide-permeated processed products in favor of unadulterated, natural organic commodities best suited to the task of bringing forth a child who will be both healthy and happy.

And rather than allow their infants to be bottle-fed on formula, they're reverting to the method nature designed for optimum nutrition—breastfeeding. As clinical nutritionist, author, and radio host Carol Simontacchi points out, "There are about one hundred elements found in breast milk that are missing from infant formula," the absence of any of which "has the potential for long-term damage to the vulnerable child."[19] But the nutritional quality of breast milk, Simontacchi observes, can vary depending on the mother's diet. For that reason, she recommends that nursing mothers, "whenever possible, choose organic meats and produce. Not only are organic foods higher in nutrient content, but they are free from the hormones and other chemicals that influence brain chemistry."

On the other hand, she notes, consumption of harmful substances, such as trans fatty acids and chemicals known to induce brain damage, such as MSG and aspartame (to be discussed in more detail in Chapter 2), can be passed on to the child through breastfeeding and should be avoided.[20]

Important Things to Avoid While Pregnant

One whiff of a beauty salon, with its chemically permeated atmosphere of sprays, polishes, and lacquers, should tell you it's no place for an infant. And when you enter such an environment while pregnant, its harmful effects are similarly as bad, if not worse, for your unborn baby. Just as you're "eating for two," you are also breathing for two. The chemicals and toxic substances you're exposed to while pregnant can directly affect your fetus. Many toxic substances, such as mercury and lead, can cross the placenta and damage your unborn baby in both obvious and subtle ways.

When you're pregnant, you should make every effort to stay away from chemicals and toxicants that can damage your unborn child, including:

- Lead dust. (See Chapter 6 for detailed information.)
- Mercury from eating fish, as well as from the vapors to which you could be exposed from a broken mercury thermometer. You should also avoid both getting any new mercury amalgam fillings and having the ones already in your mouth removed. (See Chapter 6.)
- Fumes from painting. If your home is being painted, you should stay with a friend or relative until the house is completely aerated. You should also insist that low-toxicity paint be used.
- Toxic cleaning agents. (See Chapter 5 for details and alternatives.)

- Pesticide applications, both inside and outside your home.
- Any activity that would expose you to possibly toxic fumes, such as some hobbies and certain hair and nail treatments.

Raising chemical-free kids can be a family affair—prenatally, by the mother-to-be creating a healthy physical environment for the fetus, and postnatally, by the parents passing on healthy habits through setting good examples. Keep in mind, however, that it's never too late to start, and from whatever point you do, the results are bound to benefit your family and help ensure your kids of a brighter and healthier future.

Fish: Brain Food or Brain-Damaging Food?

Since 1990, when the National Academy of Science published its seafood safety report, there have been discussions, advisory panels, reports, and calls for action about the levels of mercury in seafood. While fish should be an important part of our menu, fish that is high in mercury should be avoided or eaten sparingly, particularly if you are pregnant, nursing, trying to conceive, or feeding young children.

Further complicating the issue is the fact that the EPA standards apply only to recreationally caught fish. The FDA, which controls commercial fishing, employs standards that are generally less strict and often rely on dated data, some of it more than twenty years old. Mercury-contaminated fish is the main source of human exposure to this toxic heavy metal, with freshwater and large, long-living fish (such as shark) accumulating the highest levels. Your state should have its own advisories, based on the EPA guidelines, so before feeding any of your children fish that you or a friend may have caught, check to find out if there is any sort of advisory posted for the waters where it was caught.

Canned tuna receives a lot of attention, as it's probably the most frequently consumed fish. The Environmental Working Group, a consumer-advocacy organization in Washington, DC, is much more cautious in its recommendations for women than either the EPA or the FDA. (See "Fish Consumption Advice," from the Environmental Working Group, below.) If you can't follow its guidelines to the letter, you should still try to avoid the most contaminated fish at the top of the list, especially while pregnant. The devastating effects of mercury on fetal development, which can result from both large and small exposures, include brain damage, mental retardation, lack of coordination, blindness, and seizures. Even small fetal exposures to mercury can do lasting damage to language comprehension, memory, and the ability to focus. There is ongoing research to evaluate whether mercury exposure in utero can also contribute to learning defects as a child develops. (This subject will be explored in greater detail in Chapter 6.)

FISH CONSUMPTION ADVICE

The following advice is courtesy of the Environmental Working Group, whose Web site can be found at www.ewg.org.
Pregnant women should avoid eating:

Gulf Coast oysters	Shark
Halibut	Swordfish
King mackerel	Tilefish
Largemouth bass	Tuna, fresh and canned
Marlin	Walleye
Pike	White croaker
Sea bass	

Pregnant women should not eat more than one serving per month of:

Blue mussel	Gulf Coast blue crab
Channel catfish (wild)	Lake whitefish
Cod	Mahi mahi
Eastern oyster	Pollock
Great Lakes salmon	

When deciding what to eat, remember that these fishes are lowest in mercury and thus safe to eat at least twice a week:

Blue crab (mid-Atlantic)	Haddock
Catfish (farmed)	Salmon (wild Pacific)
Croaker	Shrimp
Flounder (summer)	Trout (farmed)

When deciding what to eat, remember that data from the 1970s (the most recent) shows that these fishes have the highest concentrations of mercury and should be avoided:

Bluefish	Porgy
Bonito	Rockfish
Lake trout	Snapper
Orange roughy	

In this chapter, we've attempted to define some of the challenges facing parents who want their kids to enjoy the benefits of physical, mental, and emotional health, and to explain why we can't rely on even the best efforts of regulators to protect us from toxic products. In the chapters that follow, we'll offer more details, both of the problems we face today in trying to safeguard our families from the pernicious effects of chemical contaminants and of the practical and effective solutions that we can put into action.

RESOURCES

Bovine Growth Hormone

Organic Consumers Association/BioDemocracy Campaign
Web site: http://organicconsumers.org/rbghlink.html
The Web site of the grassroots organization based in Little Marais, Minnesota, seeking organic, nonirradiated food for human and animal health.

Environmental Pollutants and Toxicants

Envirohealthaction
Web site: www.envirohealthaction.org/index.cfm
An education and action Web site sponsored by the Physicians for Social Responsibility, Washington, DC.

Fluoride

Citizens for Safe Drinking Water
Web site: www.nofluoride.com
Articles and studies against water fluoridation.

Fluoride: Journal of the International Society for Fluoride Research
Web site: www.fluoride-journal.com
Technical articles and studies related to the biological and other effects of fluoride on animal, plant, and human life.

Food Quality Protection Act (FQPA)

FQPA
Web site: www.ecologic-ipm.com/menu.html
Issues, resources, findings, and reports related to the implementation of the FQPA, presented by the Consumers Union of Yonkers, New York.

Natural Health Information

Citizens for Health
Web site: www.citizens.org
The Web site of the national, nonprofit grassroots organization protecting health choices.

Reproductive Toxins

Children's Environmental Health Project
Web site: http://children.cape.ca/repro.html

The Web site of the Canadian Association of Physicians for the Environment.

Generations at Risk
Web site: www.safer-world.org/e/chem/reproduc.htm
A report by the Greater Boston Physicians for Social Responsibility (GBPSR) and the Massachusetts Public Interest Research Group (MASSPIRG) Education Fund.

❋ **2** ❋

Overcoming Additive Addictions

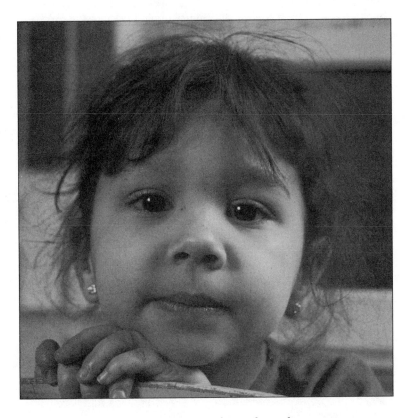

"You have the right to eat. You have the right to eat wholesome foods. You have the right to read about the foods you are about to eat."
  —John C. Stauber and Sheldon Rampton, *Toxic Sludge Is Good for You!* (Common Courage Press, 1995)

WHAT YOU'LL FIND IN THIS CHAPTER

Artificial colors come shaded with unnecessary risks. While foods imbued with natural colors are apt to contain a multitude of nutrients, the artificial dyes used to make processed products more appealing can also make them more hazardous to your family's health. Once derived chiefly from coal tar and now extracted largely from petroleum products, these artificial colors have a "shady" history, with a number of them having been taken out of circulation as health hazards by the FDA after initially being declared harmless. Researchers also found that baby rats became hyperactive and showed diminished learning ability when exposed to "real-world" combinations of coloring agents.

Flavorings and preservatives add to our daily consumption of chemicals. Those flavoring agents that can imitate the taste of just about anything are actually concocted in chemical laboratories, with most never having been tested for effects on physical or mental health. And some preservatives—most notably BHA, BHT, and TBHQ—are suspects in health and behavioral problems.

Exposure to excitotoxins can be lethal to certain brain cells. Excitotoxins are found in countless products, including flavor enhancers such as monosodium glutamate (MSG), hydrolyzed vegetable protein, and a variety of other ingredients that contain processed free glutamic acid. Research on test animals has found such additives to be capable of causing certain unprotected brain cells to die from overstimulation, which is why they've been dubbed "excitotoxins." The affected cells are located in the hypothalamus, a key area of the brain that controls hormone releases, hunger, thirst, and sleep, and emotions such as rage and aggression. Such findings of neurotoxicity resulted in MSG being taken out of baby food some years ago, but other excitotoxins have not been removed. And in recent years, a new one has become prevalent—the artificial sweetener aspartame (NutraSweet), which is used as a sugar substitute in most diet products, and which was allowed on the market despite the concerns of FDA advisers over findings that it caused brain tumors in rats.

Things You Can Do Now!

- Read labels carefully, and avoid artificial colors, flavors, and preservatives.

- Be especially wary of products that contain processed free glutamic acid—not just MSG, but in "hidden forms" such as hydrolyzed vegetable protein, sodium and calcium caseinate, autolyzed yeast, and quite often, natural flavors.
- Avoid any products that contain the artificial sweeteners aspartame or neotame, keeping in mind that they can turn up where you might least suspect them, such as in children's nutritional supplements. Diet sodas especially should not be given to children.
- When buying convenience foods (such as soups, pasta sauces, and frozen meals), choose organic varieties whenever possible.

Examine the labels on the overwhelming majority of the items in your neighborhood supermarket and you'll discover just how much the processed food industry depends on things produced in the chemist's laboratory. Many of the products are a veritable witches' brew of additives, whose unwanted side effects and potential for adverse reactions may in some cases be quite controversial and in others not really understood. They're there for numerous reasons, including making nutrient-deficient food tastier, making it more appealing, and giving it a longer shelf life. What's considered least (if at all) is the effect this cornucopia of chemical ingredients may have on consumers, in particular, the youngest ones. What follows are some of the more glaring examples.

WHEN YOUR FOOD IS ONLY FOOLING

"Special effects" may be fine for the movies, but when they're used to fool you about the food you and your family eat, that's another matter entirely. Unfortunately, when what your children see and taste is something other than what it's supposed to be—and turns out to have been concocted in a test tube—it can also affect them in ways that you might never have anticipated, and that aren't always obvious. And while the fine print on the label might tell you that you're being fooled by the food in the package, it won't tell you anything about the potential results.

True Colors Versus Artificial Ones

There's absolutely nothing wrong with a colorful diet, as long as the appearance of what you eat reflects its "true colors." That means your family is best served by foods that come in a variety of natural hues, such as fruits and vegetables. The consumption of colors in this form is highly desirable, a sure sign that your table is loaded with an abundance of fiber, essential nutrients, and antioxidants, which help prevent cancer and heart disease.

But there's a big difference between the nutritional pot of gold to which this sort of rainbow leads and the "fool's gold" found at the end of our synthetic rainbow of brightly colored processed foods. For while artificial colors may make products appear appetizing and attractive, they represent just the kind of chemical additives we should strive to avoid feeding to our children.

To cite just one example, FD&C Red Dye Number 2 was banned from the list of approved food colorings in 1976 by the FDA because it was shown to have produced a statistically significant rise in cancer in test animals—after having had its safety questioned by scientists for more than twenty years. By contrast, tomatoes get their beautiful red color from lycopene, which protects against certain cancers and keeps bad cholesterol from becoming oxidized and causing hardening of the arteries. They are also a source of vitamin C, a key antioxidant.

Red Dye Number 2 has not been the only artificial color to fall into disrepute after being long accepted and widely used. Over the years, the list has included a variety of synthetic hues, among them FD&C Violet Number 1. Once used not only in candy, cakes, drink powders, and soda, but also in the USDA's purple meat stamp, it was banned in 1976, fourteen years after a Canadian study found that half the rats that ingested it in their food developed cancerous growths. Then there was another scarlet shade, FD&C Red Number 3, which was banned from use in cosmetics and externally applied drugs after the FDA found it caused thyroid cancer in rats and other studies concluded it interferes with nerve impulses in the brain. Strangely enough, however, its use in food items such as fruit salad, gelatin, and candy continued to be allowed in what one FDA expert has referred to as a "regulatory inconsistency." (Banned entirely, however, were the "lakes" of Red Number 3. "Lakes" are the water-soluble forms of colorings, mixed either with aluminum or calcium and used to prevent leaching in things like drugs and hard candies.) It's common sense that if these artificial colors have been found to be detrimental to animals, they should certainly not be given to children.

That so many supposedly "harmless" coloring agents are found to be otherwise is hardly surprising, however, when one considers their "shady" origins and backgrounds. Consider, for instance, that many of the older dyes were manufactured from coal tar—a thick, black liquid derived from coal—and that some of those are still in use today, while many newer ones are petroleum extracts. In addition, under FDA certification rules, they may contain certain amounts of contaminants, such as lead, mercury, and arsenic.[1] These don't sound like the kinds of things you'd deliberately want to add to your family's dinner menu! Dr. Magaziner has been diagnosing more and more children with toxic levels of harmful metals, including lead and mercury, and finding a correlation with these children having problems such as autism, attention deficit disorder (ADD), and developmental delays.

Controversy and notoriety, in fact, have colored the entire history of artificial colors. It was, for example, the use of toxic substances to color and often disguise the appearance of food at the beginning of the twentieth century that brought about passage of the Pure Food and Drugs Act of 1906, the first federal food-safety law. But while that legislation may have pulled the plug on some of the most blatantly dangerous color additives, it didn't stop many other harmful ones from continuing to be used. So in 1938, it was expanded, defining how colors can be used with the addition of the FD&C designations and calling for special certification for coal tar dyes.

Simply putting more teeth in the law, however, didn't automatically result in the removal of all unhealthy hues from the market, either. It took a number of subsequent studies to determine that various color additives originally deemed "harmless" in fact weren't, along with an incident in the 1950s in which children were made ill by the artificial coloring in popcorn and candies. That led to the banning of three chemical dyes and a further reevaluation of coloring agents in 1960. But despite all that, many that are suspected health risks continue to serve as flamboyant "fronts" for all kinds of foods. Other artificial colors have been shown to trigger asthma and allergies, some attacks of which can be life-threatening.

As with pesticides, there's always the potential that mixing two or more chemical ingredients together can increase the likelihood of a toxic effect via the process known as synergy (in which the effects of the different substances are more powerful—or in this case, more toxic—when they are combined). In studies performed at Yale University's Department of Pediatric Neurology, for instance, baby rats exposed to a mixture of five artificial colors became hyperactive and showed diminished learning ability. The experiment was one that approximated the kinds of real-world dietary exposures to such substances that children are apt to experience. (It has been estimated that a child consumes, on average, some 325 milligrams of synthetic dyes daily.) "Our results provide additional support for the belief that the administration of food colorings may exert significant effects in the developing organism," the researchers concluded.[2]

While such an effect has never been decisively proven where kids are concerned, Dr. Magaziner has noticed that attention deficit and hyperactivity problems decrease when chemical additives are removed. Such observations make it all the more important for parents not to wait while the scientists debate, not when the well-being of their children is at stake. What we've already learned from the record of artificial colors is that they can't really be trusted with our families' health and, in any event, serve no purpose other than to try to fool us. Unlike the natural colors with which nature has endowed our food, artificial colors are positively worthless as indicators of nutritional value under the surface. But they may sometimes be used in an attempt to "spruce up" those natural colors without any notice to the consumer—for instance, by being sneakily added to the strawberries used to make strawberry yogurt[3] (something that would not be allowed in organic products). So if a food item looks to you like it's a bit more colorful than nature intended, that may very well be the case, even if the label says nothing about it.

YOUR OWN TRUE COLORS!

If your kids find delight in odd-colored foods, there's no reason why you can't make your own with very little trouble.

Instead of buying blue oatmeal, put a few blueberries through the blender and mix them into plain oatmeal. How about some rosy red applesauce or lemonade? Crush some pomegranate seeds and add the juice (the seeds of a pomegranate are edible, too, but for coloring purposes, just add the juice). Pomegranate juice, incidentally, has recently been found to assist cholesterol metabolism.

Not only will you be achieving the same Technicolor results without the artificial dyes, but you'll be mixing in fiber, vitamins, and antioxidants.

To add to blueberries' many other magnificent properties, it's believed that a natural substance in the fruit, anthocyanosides, kills *E. coli* bacteria. For this reason, dried blueberries are given in Sweden to treat childhood diarrhea.[4] Blueberries may also help keep your eyes healthy and protect against heart disease.

Beware of Imitations—And Letter Combinations

If it tastes like vanilla, looks like vanilla, and comes in the same kind of bottle as vanilla, it must be vanilla, right? Not quite. And if anything, the lower price for a larger amount should be a tip-off. It's vanillin, the name of a key component of natural vanilla beans, only in this case a cheap, artificial imitation of the real thing. In fact, it comes from wood pulp, a by-product of the paper-manufacturing process.[5] (Here's a good rule of thumb to keep in mind when evaluating food additives: If the source sounds distinctly unappetizing, it's best to follow your instincts and avoid it.) It's also far less costly to produce than genuine vanilla extract. But you'd never know it to look at the ingredients of many supposed "luxury" candies and confections, which include vanillin in place of vanilla.

Of course, some scientists will tell you it doesn't make any real difference, since the chemical formulations of both real vanillin and the synthetic variety are identical. However, that doesn't take into account the adverse symptoms some children and adults develop after ingesting the artificial stuff, but not upon consuming the real McCoy. The reason for that, according to Dr. Ruth Aranow of the Johns Hopkins University Department of Chemistry, is that "every chemical synthesized contains some of the materials used in the synthesis."[6] In other words, what you're getting isn't "pure," but rather a substance that comes with "extra baggage" in the form of a laboratory chemical residue that may include "high levels of sulfites and other contaminants," according to the Feingold Association of the United States (FAUS).[7] And for someone who's especially sensitive to chemicals, as a growing number of people are, that could be enough to tip the balance and produce a bad reaction (which is why the Feingold Program of dietary management for children and adults allows the use of vanilla, but not artificial vanillin).

While you can usually find vanillin next to the vanilla extract in the spice aisle of your grocery store, most of the numerous other "flavors"—substances designed to imitate the taste of something—contained in countless processed foods are things you couldn't ordinarily purchase as commodities unless you were a manufacturer. And as Eric Schlosser notes in his book *Fast Food Nation*, each of these is apt to consist, not of a single substance, but rather of a carefully concocted combination of chemicals so that "the taste of a food will be radically altered by minute changes in the flavoring mix."[8] But a key point that you as a parent might consider most significant is Jane Hersey's observation that most such flavoring chemicals have never undergone any testing to determine if they can cause cancer or birth defects—or for that matter, behavioral changes (which can also be caused by excitotoxins such as MSG and aspartame, discussed later in this chapter).

Not all additives, of course, are there to add taste or color to food. The purpose of preservatives, for instance, is to give commodities a longer shelf life, mostly by keeping the fats from becoming rancid. But three of the most commonly used—the petroleum derivatives BHA, BHT, and most recently, TBHQ—have been the focus of behavioral and health concerns.

The first two were the subjects of studies done in the early 1970s. After pregnant mice were fed these preservatives, their offspring were born with altered brain chemistry—that is, with their levels of cholinesterase and serotonin reduced by half. According to the researchers, "the affected mice weighed less, slept less and fought more than normal controls." In addition, BHA and BHT are banned or restricted in various other countries, and BHA is listed as a carcinogen by the state of California and a possible carcinogen by the World Health Organization. As for TBHQ, it has been known to cause death following ingestion of as little as 5 grams, and symptoms such as nausea and vomiting, ringing in the ears, delirium, a sense of suffocation, and collapse with ingestion of just 1 gram (a thirtieth of an ounce).[9]

Then there's the strange case of brominated vegetable oil, or BVO, which, like artificial colors, has a purely cosmetic purpose—to keep certain citrus drinks from clouding up in the bottle. Despite its harmless-sounding name, it caused heart damage in test animals used in studies conducted back in the 1960s. But when consumer advocates James S. Turner and Michael Jacobson (the latter now the director of the Center for Science in the Public Interest) sued the FDA to halt its use, a judge responded by allowing the agency to place it in the newly created category of "interim" additives that require further study before being approved or rejected. And that's where it has sat in the quarter century or so since—while continuing to be used in those citrus-based drinks.[10]

ADDITIVES THAT SHORT-CIRCUIT THE BRAIN

They're often referred to as "excitotoxins" because of their ability to literally excite brain cells to death. Are we talking about another one of those illegal drugs that kids are always being warned about? No, we're referring to certain common food additives readily available in your supermarket that, while perfectly legal, can do irreparable harm to your kids if consumed in sufficient quantities. Most notable are those containing glutamic acid, such as MSG, and aspartame, the synthetic sweetener found in so many "sugar-free" products.

Glutamic Bombs

If the phenomenal growth of processed foods has led to a corresponding rise in the use of artificial colors, flavors, and preservatives, it has also caused the use of flavor enhancers to skyrocket in recent years. These additives utilize processed free glutamic acid (as opposed to the kind that is naturally bound into food) to amplify the often bland taste of products that have been short-changed on basic ingredients or stripped of natural nutrients during processing before being frozen, canned, or vacuum sealed. Perhaps the best known of these is monosodium glutamate, or MSG, although there is a whole bevy of others contained in the products that line today's supermarket shelves, including hydrolyzed vegetable protein, sodium and calcium caseinate, and autolyzed yeast (not to mention such ingredients as "natural flavors," which may well be additional sources).

For families with kids, however, the proliferation of these additives has been most unfortunate, since they should be avoided at all cost according to some of the most respected people in the field of neuroscience. Despite reassurances by the FDA and the glutamate industry (yes, there is a glutamate industry) that reactions to MSG are mild and temporary, these experts cite research showing that excessive amounts of glutamate can have a potentially damaging effect on the still evolving brains of infants and children. It's as if much of our food contains tiny "glutamic bombs" capable of destroying brain cells in vulnerable individuals—those whose protective blood-brain barriers are either not yet fully developed or else have been damaged or compromised. Originally isolated from seaweed, MSG (along with hydrolyzed vegetable protein) was first produced and marketed as a flavor enhancer in Japan by the Ajinomoto Company, which remains the world's major supplier. As it found its way into more and more products during the 1950s and 1960s, in addition to being marketed as an off-the-shelf flavor enhancer (mostly under the trade name "Accent"), it started to acquire something of a negative reputation. After eating meals to which MSG had been liberally added, some Chinese restaurant patrons began to develop headaches and other symptoms, such as muscle fatigue, aches, and numbness. The condition even acquired a name—"Chinese restaurant syndrome." But its symptoms were largely dismissed as superficial, transient reactions.

In the meantime, researchers discovered some more alarming propensities of MSG. In 1957, two ophthalmologists tested it on infant mice to see if it could be used as a treatment for a particular condition and instead found that it destroyed nerve cells in the inner layers of the retina. A decade later, Dr. John Olney, a prominent neurosurgeon associated with Washington University in St. Louis, found it had a similar effect on cells, or neurons, in the hypothalamus, a key part of the brain that controls the release of hormones, as well as emotions like rage and aggression, hunger and thirst, and the sleep and waking cycles. In 1969, the disclosure of that information to Congress was enough to get MSG voluntarily removed from baby food, to which manufacturers had been routinely adding it in amounts equivalent to those that had produced brain damage in test animals.[11]

It might seem strange that brain damage can be inflicted by glutamic acid, a substance that actually plays a role in the brain as a neurotransmitter (sending information from neuron to neuron). But as it turns out, that's precisely what makes it a threat to brain cells when introduced in excess of what nature intended. In the presence of too much glutamate, the neurons of the hypothalamus, which are particularly receptive to glutamate and which are not shielded by the blood-brain barrier, become overexcited and fire repetitively (hence the name "excitotoxin"). Such overstimulation wreaks havoc on the cells by letting in too much calcium, which in turn triggers an influx of free radicals, which can inflict lethal cell damage.[12]

Some experts believe that feeding excitotoxins to newborns and young children can result in just this sort of damage, with potentially devastating effects on learning ability, personality, and behavior. As neurosurgeon Dr. Russell Blaylock notes in his book *Excitotoxins: The Taste That Kills* (Health Press, 1996), "Sometimes, the effects might be subtle, such as a slight case of dyslexia, or more severe, such as frequent outbursts of uncontrollable anger . . . There is a possibility that early exposure to excitotoxins could cause a tendency for episodic violence and criminal behavior in later years."[13] In light of the recent unprecedented epidemic of rage-induced mass shootings in high schools, that kind of warning takes on urgent new significance.

Such concerns, as Dr. Blaylock points out, have been amplified by experiments with mice and other animals. Injecting tiny amounts of glutamate into the hypothalamus of test animals, for instance, has been shown to produce sudden rage. In another experiment, baby rats given low doses of MSG injected under their skin became hyperactive, grew to be shorter and fatter than control animals, and had far more trouble navigating mazes.[14] Exposure to excitotoxins such as MSG has also been shown to cause early onset of puberty in female rats.[15]

The FDA's tendency has been to shut off such alarm bells by attempting to reassure the public that all is well and that MSG poses no problems for the majority of people, largely echoing the messages emanating from the Glutamate Association, made up of manufacturers and users. In doing so, it has chosen to dismiss not only the findings of prominent scientists, but countless reports of adverse reactions to MSG that run the gamut from headaches and seizures to digestive ailments. Such reactions are apparent indicators of MSG sensitivity, a condition that seems to afflict people of all ages. "MSG-sensitive people typically react to any glutamic acid that has been freed from protein through a manufacturing process, provided that they ingest amounts that exceed their tolerance to MSG," notes Jack Samuels, a spokesman for the Illinois-based Truth-in-Labeling Campaign. A possible reason, Samuels adds, is the fact that processed free glutamic acid contains "an array of contaminants" not found in the glutamic acid naturally contained in various commodities.

Unfortunately, the problem has been complicated by the use of the term "MSG" itself, since MSG is only one of the additives that might cause such reactions. In fact, the FDA, in a document issued in 1995, noted that the use of phrases such as "No added MSG" may be deceptive and misleading, since "MSG" is commonly used to refer to all free glutamic acid, but is not the only source of it. Therefore, products described as containing "no added MSG" may still contain free glutamic acid. (For a list of sources of processed free glutamic acid, see page 50.)

Whatever they're called, MSG and other forms of processed free glutamic acid are now present in so many products (even in some commercial baby foods that claim to "contain no MSG") that removing them would require sweeping and profound changes in the regulatory process. That's why it's up to you as a parent to evaluate these warnings for yourself and to hopefully eliminate as many products that contain these additives as possible from your family's diet. (If you don't have the time to prepare your own baby food, for instance, you might want to opt for commercial organic baby food, which is now widely available in most supermarkets.) It may take some vigilance, but once you get into the habit of reading the ingredients list on labels, you'll become familiar with which products to avoid. And of course, the more you prepare food in your own kitchen instead of grabbing a frozen kids' dinner or can of pasta, the safer your family will be from the potential harm inflicted by "glutamic bombs."

SOURCES OF PROCESSED FREE GLUTAMIC ACID

MSG isn't the only source of processed free glutamic acid to which people suffer adverse reactions. It's also hidden in many other ingredients.

The following additives always contain processed free glutamic acid:

Autolyzed yeast	Monopotassium glutamate
Calcium caseinate	Monosodium glutamate
Gelatin	Sodium caseinate
Glutamate	Textured protein
Glutamic acid	Yeast extract
Hydrolyzed corn gluten	Yeast food
Hydrolyzed protein	Yeast nutrient

These additives often contain processed free glutamic acid:

Anything enzyme modified	Natural pork flavoring
Anything fermented	Pectin
Anything protein fortified	Protease
Barley malt	Protease enzymes
Bouillon	Seasonings
Broth	Soy protein
Carrageenan	Soy protein concentrate
Enzymes (any kind)	Soy protein isolate
Flavors and flavorings	Soy sauce
Malt extract	Soy sauce extract
Malt flavoring	Stock
Maltodextrin	Whey protein
Natural beef flavoring	Whey protein concentrate
Natural chicken flavoring	Whey protein isolate
Natural flavors and flavorings	

FAKE FOOD CITATION
Instant Noodle Soup

Wow, is this easy, and kids just love those noodles! In just about four minutes, you can serve your kids 770 milligrams of sodium; monosodium glutamate; hydrolyzed corn, soy, and wheat protein (more sources of processed free glutamic acid); autolyzed yeast extract (yet another form); partially hydrogenated vegetable oil; and so much more!

The brand we saw proclaims that the noodles make not only "exciting" soups, but a better salad. The "exciting" part is certainly true, when you consider that one of the ingredients added to it is the excitotoxin MSG, which can literally "excite" brain cells to death. (Studies have shown that MSG in liquids such as soups is absorbed faster and is much more toxic to the brain than MSG in solid food.[16]) While soup can make a wonderfully nutritious meal for kids (and can serve as a great vehicle for lots of different vegetables), fake soup is worse than nothing. And what a shame to adulterate a perfectly healthy salad.

If soup is on your menu, your health-food store offers far better ready-to-serve varieties without all the artificial ingredients. If your kids love noodles, you can add them. Or better yet, dust off the crockpot and make some vegetable soup. It's easier than you think.

The Not-So-Sweet Sweetener

You don't have to be a nutritionist to know that refined sugar isn't particularly good for kids. Besides helping to promote tooth decay, it's known to produce a spike in blood sugar, to which the body responds with a burst of insulin—a form of internal stress. It also causes a "high" that's soon followed by a "low"—that is, a period of lethargy (which, considering how many sugary snacks and drinks are available in school, may be one reason why kids become inattentive in class). In addition, some experts consider table sugar, or sucrose, to be a deterrent to healthy physical and mental development because of the "empty calories" it substitutes for vital nutrients and, along with fructose (a sugar derived

from fruit and used extensively in soft drinks in the form of high
fructose corn syrup), to cause depletion of the essential trace ele-
ment chromium.

HIGH-FRUCTOSE CORN SYRUP: WHAT IS IT?

While refined sugar was once the sweetener found in most processed
foods and drinks, since the 1970s a cheaper alternative—high-
fructose corn syrup (HFCS)—has become the sweetener of choice
in practically all soft drinks as well as in many other products.
Produced by treating corn syrup with enzymes to make it sweeter,
HFCS can now be found in all sorts of conventional processed
foods, even dog foods!

While fructose generally does not produce a high insulin response (it is metabolized differently from other simple sugars),
HFCS does produce this response and hence has a very high
glycemic index. (The glycemic index is a way to measure how
quickly certain foods are likely to raise your blood sugar.) In other
words, HFCS can rapidly increase your blood sugar—and hence
your insulin—level, which is particularly ill-advised in diabetics and
those with hypoglycemia.

Another problem with HFCS (and this includes regular fructose
as well) is that it can trigger the loss of chromium, an essential
trace mineral, according to Richard Anderson, lead scientist with
the U.S. Department of Agriculture Human Nutrition Research
Center in Beltsville, Maryland. According to Anderson, low chromium
levels can play a role in anything that's related to insulin, including
diabetes, hypoglycemia, obesity, hypertension, cardiovascular disease, and even eye and nerve problems.[17]

Before you offer your family fruit juice as a healthy alternative to
soda, however, look at the ingredients. It, too, may well be sweetened with HFCS. Your best bet: organic, 100 percent fruit juice that
is not from concentrate. And don't forget water, which is healthy
and inexpensive, provided that the impurities and toxic substances, including fluoride, have been filtered out. Diet soda, which
is sweetened with aspartame, is not a healthful substitute for soda
containing HFCS.

Many soft drinks are loaded with sugar, some containing up to 10 teaspoons for every 12 ounces of soda. Put this together with the fact that kids often drink two or three cans of soda per day, and it could well help to account for the apparent increase in cases of "attention deficit disorder." But substituting "sugar-free" products, rather than alleviating ADD and aggressive behavior, is only apt to make them worse.

In a University of Wisconsin study, for instance, some 154 male teenagers, the majority of them considered delinquents, were divided into two groups, one of which was given breakfast cereal with a high sugar content while the other was given cereal sweetened with a placebo. Before and after they ate, both groups were given neuropsychological tests for such factors as hyperactivity, concentration, mood, and behavioral disturbances. The researchers concluded that the worst-behaved subjects actually performed better in the tests after being fed the sugary cereal than the ones who got the placebo, and that the nondelinquents in the sugar-eating group also rated better in mood and behavior.[18]

Those results may sound like vindication for sugar (which is certainly the way nutritionist and author Jean Carper interpreted them) until you consider what was in those placebos. It was the artificial sweetener aspartame, a substance implicated in thousands of reports of adverse reactions (and blamed for untold numbers that have gone unreported) and is believed by some experts in neurology to pose a threat to the healthy development of children's brains. Rather than exonerating white sugar, the experiment may have unwittingly provided further evidence of aspartame's harmful effects.

It's unfortunate that an ill-advised and apparently politically motivated FDA approval, together with a multimillion-dollar barrage of soothing corporate literature, has largely succeeded in misrepresenting aspartame as a safe and wholesome sugar substitute. As a result of that, and the fact that aspartame is now the test-tube sweetener of choice in most "diet" and "sugar-free" products, many people mistakenly believe they're doing what's best for their family's health by purchasing it. But as that University of

Wisconsin study indicated, its effects could actually be considerably worse, especially for children, than those of plain old sugar. Interestingly, some of the most damaging evidence against aspartame came from a two-year safety study conducted by G. D. Searle, the original manufacturer of NutraSweet, prior to its approval in 1981. The study used 320 rats that were given aspartame and a control group of 120 that weren't. When it was over, 12 of the aspartame-fed rats had developed brain tumors (which afflicted none in the control group), with the most tumors appearing in the rats fed the highest doses of aspartame. In any event, by the company's own estimate, that figure was twenty-five times higher than the number of rats that would ordinarily be expected to develop spontaneous brain tumors.

However, when Dr. Olney, the MSG researcher, reviewed other rat studies, he found it was more like forty-seven times higher. He also found that brain tumors in rats are extremely rare before the age of one and a half years (seventy-eight weeks), yet five of those fed aspartame had developed them by the age of seventy weeks. And since the rate at which such tumors grow accelerates sharply after rats reach two years of age, he determined that there probably would have been many more had the Searle study not stopped at that precise point.

Dr. Olney's discoveries came about after he attempted to review the test results with the FDA's Aspartame Board of Inquiry, only to be told that they represented spontaneous brain-tumor development. This led to further studies by Searle, which found roughly equal numbers of brain tumors in both rats fed aspartame and ones that weren't, but both at a rate thirty times higher than the accepted figure. Serious doubts were later shed on these strange results, however, when an FDA investigation of Searle's laboratories turned up "apparent irregularities in data collection and reporting practices."[19]

While brain tumors might have been the biggest source of worry regarding aspartame (and in fact, the type reported in the rats has reportedly increased by more than 10 percent in recent years in humans of all ages and by 67 percent in those over sixty-five), there have been other concerns as well. By feeding aspartic acid, a key aspartame component, to rats, for instance, Dr. Olney discovered it produced microscopic holes in their brains. But then, as neurosurgeon Dr. Russell Blaylock points out, aspartic acid (or aspartate), like the glutamic acid in MSG, is an excito-toxin, a neurotransmitter capable of exciting brain cells to death if given to children in large enough doses.[20]

Another pernicious aspect of aspartame is that it breaks down into methanol, or wood alcohol, in the gut, especially when it's heated—a factor that may be responsible for the many claims of eye problems, ranging from blurred vision to blindness, that have resulted from its use. (Although many theories abound for Gulf War syndrome among veterans, one is that the decomposition of the aspartame in diet soda exposed to the desert heat may have been a cause.)

Especially affected have been airline pilots, hundreds of whom have reportedly called a special hot-line number installed by the Aspartame Consumer Safety Network, a Dallas-based organization (see "Resources" at the end of this chapter). Some have reported having harrowing experiences as a result of seizure episodes and vision problems that immediately followed the consumption of "diet" drinks, which are loaded with aspartame.[21]

Then there's that other aspartame ingredient, phenylalanine, also an amino acid and a neurotransmitter responsible for the only label warning associated with aspartame, one directed toward people suffering from a rare genetic metabolic disorder known as phenylketonuria (PKU). That, however, may not be the only problem associated with it. Some experts believe that it can also reduce levels of serotonin, a mood-enhancing chemical, in the brains of susceptible individuals.[22] If that's true, consumption of things like diet soda could well bring about depression, anxiety, and related problems for some people.

The FDA, of course, is well aware of aspartame's highly questionable safety record, having been on the receiving end of thousands of complaints about all kinds of adverse reactions to it (as have various consumer groups, including the Aspartame Consumer Safety Network), many involving migraines and seizures. These have not all been merely unsubstantiated claims. When they were initially investigated by the U.S. Centers for Disease Control (CDC), the presence of such symptoms was found to correspond with aspartame use in at least a quarter of cases.[23]

Despite all of that, aspartame has become so entrenched in the marketplace as a sweetener in countless products that its use is unlikely to be restricted anytime soon. That's why, as in the case of MSG, avoiding it (as parents by all means should do) calls for exercising particular vigilance to make sure it doesn't inadvertently sneak into the family diet. The presence of this synthetic sweetening agent in a food item isn't always noted with a swirling NutraSweet symbol. It may simply be listed as an ingredient on a product like yogurt (especially since aspartame is now generically manufactured). Worse yet, it's often hidden among the ingredients in children's nutritional supplements and pharmaceuticals, so be sure and check the labels on these products carefully before bringing them home. (Fortunately, children's nutritional supplements sold in health-food stores rarely contain aspartame.)

What about neotame, the newest artificial sweetener on the market, a close relative of aspartame, only sweeter and more concentrated? Is it safer to consume? Critics were quick to denounce its approval by the FDA in July 2002, claiming that tests on both animals and humans (funded by Monsanto, the company that developed this particular product) were inadequate and inconclusive. Comments received by the FDA included that the premarket studies produced enough negative results to indicate the need for far more extensive testing before making a decision to allow it in various products (including soft drinks). Among their points of concern were unexplained growth deficiencies in test animals, the company's explanations for which were supposedly not supported by the experimental data submitted. In addition, limited studies with Type II diabetics may show evidence of adverse effects on glycemic control, described in one analysis as "quite worrisome."

Another unresolved issue is the possibility that neotame may cause the formation of nitrosamine compounds, which can have toxic or carcinogenic effects on the liver. This was but one of the concerns expressed in a detailed report submitted to the FDA by a law firm representing an unidentified party who, quite obviously, was intimately acquainted with the research and its implications.

Given the fact that similar doubts were raised regarding the validity of the studies on aspartame, which ultimately proved to have adverse effects on many people, it would probably be wise to be wary of this newest—and largely untested—drug on the sweetener market. Unless, of course, you find it an appealing idea to let your family be used as guinea pigs.

As for sweetening your family's food, that need not involve having to choose between refined sugar and aspartame (or neotame). There are natural sweeteners out there that are far more desirable than sugar in terms of nutritional value and that are metabolized more slowly, creating less of an insulin response. They include brown rice syrup, barley malt, pure maple syrup, date sugar, less refined forms of sugar cane such as Sucanat, and of course, honey (although raw honey is not recommended for infants because of a small risk of botulism). Or for a natural, noncaloric sugar substitute, there's stevia, an herb used for many centuries by South American Indians and now consumed all over the world with no evidence that it causes adverse reactions. Available in the United States as a dietary supplement, it is reputed to stabilize blood sugar and to actually help prevent tooth decay (although these claims, it should be noted, are not officially supported by the FDA). For a detailed listing of the naturally sweet alternatives to sugar and their pros and cons, see Table 2.1.

TABLE 2.1
Naturally Sweet Alternatives to Sugar

Sweetener	Description	Disadvantages
Barley malt	Barley malt is created when fermenting bacteria in the grain turns its starch into sugars, mostly maltose. The final product is more of a "whole food" than some other sweeteners. Barley malt powder tastes like a mildly sweet malted milk ball. Because it's not as sweet as sugar, you may need to add up to 50% more in recipes.	Barley malt is a little higher in calories than sugar—120 calories per ¼ cup, compared to 95 calories per ¼ cup for refined sugar.
Brown rice syrup	Brown rice syrup is brown rice that has been ground, cooked, and mixed with enzymes that change the starch into maltose. It tastes like moderately sweet butterscotch and can be quite delicious. In recipes, you may have to use up to 50% more than you would sugar, while reducing the amount of other liquids. The sweetener is also sold as a dried powder.	Calorie-wise, ¼ cup of brown rice syrup contains 170, while 1 ½ teaspoons of the powder contain 25 (a bit more than sugar).

Sweetener	Description	Disadvantages
Date sugar	Date sugar is not sugar, but rather finely ground dates containing all of the fruit's nutrients and minerals. If you like the taste of dates, this will definitely appeal to you. Date sugar can be used as a direct replacement for sugar in cooking, although it's a bit expensive.	Date sugar will not dissolve in beverages and is best used in baking.
Fructose	Fructose can be extracted from fruits, but it is typically refined from corn. It does not cause a dramatic blood-sugar rise because it is metabolized differently from other simple sugars. It is much sweeter than sugar, so less can be used.	Fructose is known to stimulate chromium and copper loss. The USDA has also reported adverse effects on laboratory animals.
Honey	Honey is one of the oldest natural sweeteners on the market. It is sweeter than sugar and has different flavors depending on the plant source. Some are very dark and intensely flavored. Raw honey contains small amounts of enzymes, minerals, and vitamins. When replacing sugar with honey in a recipe, reduce the amounts of other liquids.	Honey is higher in calories than sugar and high on the glycemic index. There is a small risk of botulism from giving raw honey to infants under one year old, which is why it should never be fed to them.

Sweetener	Description	Disadvantages
Maple syrup	Maple syrup adds a nice flavor to foods, but it is probably not a good idea to replace all the sweeteners in a recipe with it. Make sure you buy 100 percent pure maple syrup, not maple-flavored corn syrup. Organic varieties are also available.	Maple syrup is high in calories and high on the glycemic index. There has been concern about possible chemical additives in U.S. products, so some people prefer Canadian brands or organically produced maple syrup.
Molasses	Organic molasses is probably the most nutritious sweetener derived from sugar cane. Different types of molasses have different flavors, but most impart a very distinctive taste. Use less molasses than you would sugar.	Molasses is high in calories. If you're not crazy about the taste, mix it with other sweeteners in your recipes.
Organic cane	Florida Crystals is a brand name for a line of less-refined cane sweeteners, including ones made from organic sugar cane. The company makes no claims related to the products' nutritional values.	Though less refined than table sugar, these products are still sugar.
Stevia	Stevia is an herb native to South America that is noncaloric and sweeter than sugar. It comes in several forms, including finely ground leaves,	Using too much powdered stevia imparts a bitter taste. Stevia cannot be replaced with sugar on a cup-for-cup basis. If you want to

Sweetener	Description	Disadvantages
	dried leaves, liquid concentrate, and white concentrate powder. White stevia powder is about 300 times sweeter than sugar, so you would use very little. The FDA allows stevia to be sold only as a dietary supplement with no mention of sweetness on the package.	cook with it, your best bet is to get a stevia cookbook and follow the measurements carefully. Stevia also combines very well with other natural sweeteners.
Sucanat	Sucanat is a brand name for an organic evaporated cane-juice product that has been blended with organic molasses. Sucanat looks like coarse brown beach sand and has a very mild, brown sugar-like taste. It can be used as a cup-for-cup replacement for white sugar.	Sucanat has slightly more calories than white sugar, but retains more of the vitamins and minerals of the sugar cane.
Turbinado sugar	Turbinado sugar is very coarse and crunchy. It's evaporated cane juice that has been less refined than white sugar. A good way to use turbinado sugar is to sprinkle some on top of a dish such as homemade cookies or apple sauce. Because of its coarse nature, it doesn't dissolve too easily and gives a sweet taste without too much being used.	Turbinado sugar is less processed than refined white sugar, but is still sugar.

THE FEINGOLD FORMULA FOR KEEPING KIDS OFF RITALIN

For some kids, the need to become "chemical-free" is a lot more urgent than for others. They're the ones whose disruptive behavior, learning difficulties, or inability to interact may well be triggered by dietary factors, especially hypersensitivity to or intolerance for even tiny amounts of certain specific food additives.

The relationship between a child's behavior and performance and what he or she eats is a concept whose critical importance is starting to be acknowledged by a growing number of medical professionals—but is still unfamiliar territory to many others. As a result, a youngster may often be labeled as a "problem child" and administered a medication such as Ritalin, Adderall, Concerta, or Prozac. The medication may then well lead to new psychological problems or even drug dependency, when all the child really needs is to stop eating whatever it is that's actually causing the hyperactivity, belligerence, lack of cooperation, or inability to concentrate.

Fortunately, children who suffer from such syndromes can get the kind of help they really need by becoming part of a highly acclaimed and successful program, one aimed at identifying and eliminating the elements in a child's (or adult's) diet that may be acting as impediments to his or her development.

The Feingold Program is the result of work done by the late Dr. Benjamin F. Feingold, a pediatrician and chief of allergy at the Kaiser Permanente Medical Center in San Francisco. He was considered a pioneer in the fields of allergy and immunology, and is best known for making the connection between what we eat and how it affects the way we feel and behave. Since 1976, his work has been continued by a nonprofit organization of parents and professionals called the Feingold Association of the United States.

The association's program eliminates several groups of synthetic additives: synthetic food dyes; artificial flavorings; synthetic sweeteners such as aspartame, neotame, saccharine, and cyclamates; and three preservatives, BHA, BHT, and TBHQ. At the start of the program, salicylates are also removed, but may be added back and tested one at a time. Foods high in naturally occurring salicylates include apples, oranges, tomatoes, and grapes. (Aspirin is also a source.) The salicylates can be reintroduced and tested after four to six weeks.

The association researches brand-name foods to identify which ones are free of the offending additives and natural salicylates. It also provides comprehensive information and support to guide families through the program. Food-list books include thousands of acceptable products for seven different regions of the United States. Monthly newsletters provide updates on new products that can be added, and alerts about ones that have been changed and should be avoided. Even fast food restaurants are researched. One of the advantages of the Feingold Program is that parents can test it out in their home, using ordinary foods available in their neighborhood supermarket. It allows children to continue to eat most of the things they enjoy, seeking to eliminate from their diet only those that contain ingredients that might be producing their adverse reactions.

Behavioral symptoms targeted by the Feingold Program include such indicators of hyperactivity as excessive wiggling, running, and inability to sit still; impulsive and compulsive actions that are apt to be unpredictable, disruptive, destructive, or abusive; and emotional problems such as depression, irritability, panic, mood swings, and oversensitivity. Learning and developmental symptoms addressed by the program include various indicators of a short attention span, neuromuscular problems, and cognitive and perceptual disturbances, such as difficulty in recalling what is seen or heard. Physical symptoms, including sleep problems, bed-wetting, stomachaches, hives, and headaches, may also be a result of sensitivity to food additives.[24]

A more comprehensive understanding of the Feingold Program and the ways in which it can help children whose problems may be related to dietary and environmental factors can be gained by reading *Why Can't My Child Behave?* by Jane Hersey (Pear Tree

Press, 2002) or *Total Health Handbook* by Allan Magaziner, D.O. (Kensington Books, 2000).

So before you go the Ritalin route with your child and add yet another potentially harmful chemical to those he or she is already ingesting, you might try contacting the Feingold Association (see "Resources" at the end of this chapter).

As an adjunct or alternative to the Feingold Diet, Dr. Magaziner strongly urges parents to consult with a nutritionally oriented physician who is familiar with the impact of food sensitivities and nutritional biochemistry on ADD and learning disabilities. Hundreds of his patients have improved after their specific food allergies were identified and treated. He also recommends a thorough evaluation of nutritional imbalances, including those involving minerals such as magnesium, zinc, copper, chromium, calcium, and manganese; amino acids; essential fatty acids; and organic acids.

Dr. Magaziner has also found that stool testing can be a valuable diagnostic tool for kids with concentration and learning difficulties. Oftentimes, he has noted an imbalance of intestinal bacteria, known as intestinal dysbiosis; an overgrowth of intestinal yeast and related organisms; the presence of intestinal parasites; or a condition known as leaky gut syndrome. If any of these conditions exist, addressing the problem will frequently be essential to seeing clinical improvement.

Of course, not every patient needs all of these studies; their use needs to be determined on a case-by-case basis. Every patient is an individual and needs to be treated as such.

For referrals to nutritionally oriented physicians, contact the American Academy of Environmental Medicine or the American College for Advancement in Medicine (see "Resources" at the end of this chapter).

It's all very simple when you think about it. To help sell their products and make them more competitive, the food companies have doused them with cosmetics—a whole bevy of chemicals to make them seem more appealing. But despite their assurances that these chemicals are harmless in the quantities used, a little knowledge of what they actually are, and of their cumulative effect on health, should be enough to make them taboo in your home. Admittedly, avoiding them isn't always easy, but with a little conscientious effort, you'll soon discover that giving your family foods the way nature intended them isn't all that difficult—and can prove immensely gratifying when you realize how important it is to your kids' physical and mental health.

RESOURCES

Calorie-Free Alternatives to Artificial Sweeteners

Stevia: All About the Herb That's Sweeter Than Sugar
Web site: www.stevia.net
Studies, articles, recipes, and information about the sweet herb stevia.

Feingold Program
The Feingold Association
127 East Main Street
Suite 106
Riverhead, NY 11901
Telephone: 800-321-3287
Web site: www.feingold.org
Information about and help with the Feingold Program.

MSG and Other Excitotoxins
Aspartame Consumer Safety Network
Web site: http://web2.iadfw.net/marystod
Case studies, articles, and reports on the dangers of aspartame.

Aspartame Consumption Is Never Safe
Web site: www.aspartame.com

Information, links, and articles about the dangers of aspartame.

Battling the MSG Myth
Web site: www.msgmyth.com
A Web site that helps identify excitotoxins in food and teaches how to avoid them.

Holistic Healing Web Page
Web site: www.holisticmed.com
Articles, documents, news, and links related to holistic and alternative medicine.

No MSG
Web site: www.nomsg.com
An educational resource about the dangers of monosodium glutamate from the National Organization Mobilized to Stop Glutamate.

Say "No" to Aspartame
Web site: www.dorway.com
An educational Web site devoted to the dangers of aspartame.

The Truth-in-Labeling Campaign
Web site: www.truthinlabeling.org
One of the most complete MSG-information sites on the Web.

Physician Referrals

American Academy of Environmental Medicine (AAEM)
7701 East Kellogg
Suite 625
Wichita, KS 67207
Telephone: 316-684-5500
Web site: www.aaem.com
Referrals to nutritionally oriented physicians.

American College for Advancement in Medicine (ACAM)
23121 Verdugo Drive
Suite 204
Laguna Hills, CA 92653
Telephone: 800-532-3688
Web site: www.acam.org
    Referrals to nutritionally oriented physicians.

Chemical-Free Strategies

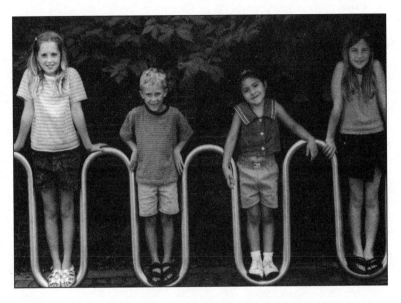

"Technology has so advanced, or retreated, depending upon one's view, that some foods are almost pure ersatz."
—Ruth Winter, M.S., *A Consumer's Dictionary of Food Additives*, Fifth Edition (Three Rivers Press, 1999)

WHAT YOU'LL FIND IN THIS CHAPTER

Good eating habits are established in early childhood. And it may surprise you to discover how much of the conventional wisdom you may have taken for granted on this subject doesn't necessarily hold up.

Two of the healthiest foods out there you won't find advertised on television. They're coconut oil, which was given an undeservedly "bad rap" until recently, and kefir, the cultured dairy product with extraordinary benefits.

Even good foods can be bad for certain children. As a parent, you should know the signs that your child might be adversely reacting to a certain type of food, particularly one that he or she is particularly fond of or in the habit of eating regularly. In this chapter, you'll learn what to look for. And you'll also learn about the role that the overuse of antibiotics can play in making children more sensitive to various foods.

Things You Can Do Now!

- Quit all this "playing around" with breakfast. It's a serious meal and one you can take charge of by replacing those sugar-and-additive-laden cereals that have turned it into playtime with the kinds of truly nutritious foods that will get your family's day off to a really good start.
- Take simple steps to free your family from exposure to harmful substances. These steps can be easily accomplished and include things such as adding one healthy food a week to their diet while reducing their consumption of processed foods, and purging their environment of pesticides and toxic chemicals.
- Our list of the ten best foods for kids can help guide you in making the transition to a healthier diet that's relatively free of chemicals and additives.
- Ten ways of introducing healthier foods to "picky eaters" can help ease that transition, by making new foods more acceptable to them and putting to rest some outdated ideas on how kids should be fed, such as forcing them into conventional mealtime routines and insisting that they clean their plates before leaving the table.

Understanding the various aspects of a problem is an important first step on the road to solving it. But unless you're ready to translate your knowledge into some form of action, "knowing better" is apt to prove only an exercise in frustration. Fortunately, there are things you can begin doing immediately to wean your children away from the pernicious influence of harmful chemicals in both their diet and their environment. These things do not involve dramatic changes in your lifestyle, but rather can be accomplished a little bit at a time. Remember, every small improvement you make is another step toward raising healthier and happier kids (and becoming a healthier and happier parent as well).

THINGS YOU CAN DO WITHOUT FURTHER ADO

Want to get your family started down the road to a less toxic lifestyle, even while you're still in the process of reading this book? Here are some suggestions.

Take Charge of Breakfast

Breakfast, as it is eaten in today's world, is all too often the worst way to start the day, particularly for kids, who have become the prime consumers of a variety of sugar-and-additive-laden excuses for cereal. But by devoting a little extra time to the effort, it's a meal you can take charge of—and one that can be a great starting point for ridding your family's diet of harmful substances. So rather than just carrying a cup of coffee with you around the house as you get yourself and your kids together for the outside world, take some time to prepare and eat a serious, healthful breakfast! Doing so will be a significant move in the direction of improving your family's health and well-being. (And if breakfast time is already an established routine in your house, you're that much ahead of the game.)

It may be a cliché, but breakfast *is* the most important meal of the day. Not only does a decent breakfast provide the energy (and brain power) necessary to get going, but kids who don't eat breakfast (and up to 30 percent of eight- to thirteen-year-olds don't), or who eat one high in sugar, are more prone to start snacking on junk food as their energy levels drop long before lunch. By contrast, studies have shown that kids who eat a real breakfast do better on school tests, have better concentration, and demonstrate improved all-around school performance. So whatever you do, don't underestimate the value of breakfast in getting the day off to a good start.

Above all, leave enough time to make breakfast for your family, rather than allowing them to fend for themselves. It can be made to jibe with how much time you have available. Running late? Go for a smoothie or an unrefined, whole-grain (and preferably organic) dry cereal. Got a few minutes to spare? Opt for eggs or hot cereal—they're well worth the little bit of extra effort. If you realize the importance of breakfast (especially for kids), you will always find time for it.

Breakfast Bummers

A close examination of some very popular breakfast choices for kids shows how giving in to marketing malarkey can start their day off all wrong.

Plenty of Nothing. The boxes are beautiful, and some of the cartoon mascots have been around for decades. But what's inside appears to be the result of a loophole in what one company calls a "commitment" to provide "you and your family with nutritious products for a healthier life."

In addition to corn, wheat, and oat flour, many commercially manufactured cereals also contain partially hydrogenated oils, which are sources of artery-gumming trans fats; artificial colors that include Yellow Number 6 and Blue Number 2, both petroleum derivatives that can produce unpleasant reactions; and the artificial preservative BHT, which can trigger allergic reactions and may be carcinogenic. (In 1972, researchers at Loyola University noted that the offspring of mice fed BHT experienced chemical changes in their brains as well as abnormal behavior patterns.) Some cereals, unfortunately, also contain modified corn starch and gelatin (which wouldn't be suitable on a vegetarian diet, as gelatin is produced by boiling animal parts—skin, tendons, bones, or ligaments—in water), along with refined flour, which contains almost no beneficial fiber and has been devitalized of most of its vitamins and minerals. Mix all that together with lots of sugar (usually in the top four of the ingredient list), and you can see this is hardly what nature intended to "break the fast" of eight hours' sleep.

Not So Hot. It takes a heap of marketing skill to turn a good breakfast food like oatmeal into a sugary (with even more grams of sugar per serving than a leading dry cereal), artificially colored, partially hydrogenated, artificially flavored, starch-containing product. One brand has even been called one of the most successful kids' foods ever introduced by its manufacturer.[1]

Adults who eat oatmeal for its health benefits may think this is a good way to introduce it to kids, and in fact, kids' oatmeal products appeal to parents because they are "healthy, convenient, and educational," according to an industry report.[2] But if you want "healthy," there are plenty of choices (including unadulterated oatmeal) that are convenient as well, and as far as "educational" goes, you can do a lot better than the "poem" on the back of one box: "Dinosaurs ruled as we all learned in school, 'til a meteor fell with great fury . . ."

It's just as easy to choose healthful, nutritious, whole-grain cereals that are high in fiber and important nutrients while low in (or devoid of) sugar and artificial ingredients.

Tips for Taking Charge of Breakfast

- Make sure you make time to eat after arising. Since an extra fifteen minutes in the morning can often make the crucial

difference, do whatever you can before bed that can save
you fifteen minutes or so when you get up, and use the time
for a sit-down breakfast instead.

- There's no law saying that breakfast must consist of cereal
or egg dishes. In Japan, breakfast might be a rice dish, and in
Mexico, beans. Often dinner leftovers make a quick (and
nutritious) breakfast. You can also consider fresh fruit or organic yogurt for breakfast.

- Smoothies are an excellent quick breakfast idea. You can
blend fruits with yogurt or milk and also add a small amount
of flaxseed oil for essential fatty acids. Kefir, a cultured milk
product, also makes an excellent smoothie base. Kefir has
beneficial intestinal bacteria (like yogurt, but in more abundance), which is why it's called a probiotic.

- Don't let kids have caffeine-containing beverages such as
coffee, tea, or cola. (Hey, they're hyper enough already!)

Ten More Steps Toward Healthier Living
You Can Take Right Now

It's easy to fall into a rut, and once you've stayed in one for a
while, it can start to feel as if you've lost the ability to climb out,
or to extricate your family. Often, however, it's the little things
you do—the little footholds—that can help you break out of your
rut and put you firmly back in command of your environment.
That's especially true when making the transition from living
under the influence of toxic chemicals to a healthier and more
wholesome existence. Here are some additional ways you can escape the rut of simply accepting whatever the chemical culture
dishes out.

Introduce Your Family to One New Healthy
Food Each Week

Pick a naturally nutritious item—be it a fruit, vegetable, grain,
or whatever (preferably organic)—that you've never served be-

fore, and integrate it into your weekly menu. Serve the food in a variety of ways, if possible. It's a chance to be creative in the kitchen while gradually enhancing your family's health and well-being. Add something new every week, and you'll find other healthy changes falling into place as you go along.

If You Don't Want Your Kids to Eat It, Don't Buy It

No matter how much whining goes on in the store, you are still the master of what goes into the grocery cart. Of course, if your kids are old enough to be making purchases on their own, you won't be able to monitor everything they eat. However, there's no reason to encourage bad eating habits, and if you've got toddlers in the house, there's no reason for them to be eating anything that you don't want them to.

Purge Your House of the Worst Offenders

While you can't change everything at once, there are certain substances that are especially harmful to kids that you should make a point of eliminating pronto. These include:

- Insecticides and herbicides
- "Diet" products that contain aspartame or neotame
- All foods that contain processed free glutamic acid in its various disguises (for a list of the various disguises, see page 50)

Make Your Own "Fast Food"

Making healthy food at home that mimics the appearance of the additive-laden ersatz entrées sold at fast food franchises is easy. The best part is that your versions will consist of actual, nutritious food, made with good ingredients that any kid will love. See Chapter 8 for some yummy suggestions.

FAKE FOOD CITATION
Colorful Little Boxes of Nonfood

The best part of these products is their exorbitant price, which might make cost-conscious parents think twice before buying them. In the United States alone, sales of these plastic trays containing small amounts of chemical-laden "food" substances comprised mainly of salt and fat have totaled more than $1.6 billion. One brand even urges kids to "make fun of lunch."

Their success can be largely attributed to pressured parents who don't have the time to pack a school lunch, giving processed-food manufacturers a chance to jump in with colorful, gimmicky concoctions that have little or no food value.

Since only 2 percent of U.S. kids go home for lunch (by contrast, in Germany, almost all children eat lunch at home, and in Italy, almost 70 percent do), the market for a no-work lunch box is gigantic.

A look at one reveals 26 grams of fat, a whopping 1,100 milligrams of sodium (and that's just from a tiny tray containing 4.8 ounces of chips and liquid "cheese"), monosodium glutamate, Yellow Numbers 5 and 6, partially hydrogenated oils, sugar, and numerous preservatives and artificial flavors.

But once in a while, can it hurt to simply give in to a popular trend? Unfortunately, it can. Aside from possible allergic and hyperactive reactions to the artificial flavorings and colors, and to the MSG, which should be avoided at all costs in children's food (see Chapter 2), there's the danger that kids who eat these ersatz, over-salted, overflavored foods may develop a taste for them. And that would really be making fun of lunch . . . and breakfast . . . and dinner.

Opt for Whole-Grain Foods Whenever Possible

Instead of white rice, go for brown rice. Instead of white bread, try whole-grain bread. Making your own pizza crust? Use whole-wheat flour instead of white flour. Little substitutions here and there will start to add up and eventually make a significant difference in your family's diet.

Cut Down on Processed Products

You might not think of fruit as being processed, but it is if it's been canned or frozen. As a rule, the more a food is processed, the less nutritious it is. Missing along with the nutrients is the taste, which is why artificial flavors are routinely added to processed foods. A canned peach doesn't taste even remotely like its fresh relative. Food was meant to be purchased fresh and consumed in a timely manner. (In many countries, for example, day-old bread is still considered stale and reduced accordingly in price, whereas in our society, packaged bread is designed to stay on the shelf for weeks.) So whenever you can, opt to buy really fresh fruits and vegetables (again, preferably organic), and if available, same-day-baked bread without preservatives. Besides being a lot better for your family, you'll find they're a whole lot tastier.

Set an Example for Your Kids

If you sit in front of the television munching chips or cookies, so will your kids. Slice some fruit and serve it with nuts (dry roasted or prepared without seasonings, which almost always contain MSG) for television snacks. Don't succumb to the ten-dollar bag of munchies at the movie theater. If you follow your own advice, your kids are more likely to do so, too.

Purify Your Family's Water

For something that's fundamental to life itself, we don't give our water much attention. What comes out of the tap is usually thought of as suitable for drinking and cooking. But water can come from many places and can be contaminated by both bacteria and numerous chemicals, some deliberately added, some not. Does your water come from a well or a municipal source? What about the condition of the pipes used to deliver it? Has your water been tested recently?

The best way to ensure high-quality water for drinking and cooking is to either install a water purification system in your home or buy purified water from a reliable source. A home system can filter just the kitchen tap or the entire house.

The cheapest and most popular method is to use a carbon block. Remember, however, that carbon will not remove fluoride or heavy metals from your water. Also, carbon filters need to be changed regularly.

Other methods of water purification include distillation and reverse osmosis, both of which remove fluoride, heavy metals, and asbestos, but not chlorine. (Reverse osmosis will also remove numerous pesticides and organic chemicals.) If these home systems are over your budget, you can still purchase water purified by these methods at your supermarket or health-food store. Just be sure to use a hard plastic container—not the soft, pliable kind—for storage. You might also consider having spring water delivered to your home in glass jugs. (Glass is still the best container for liquids, especially water and oil.) It's well worth the added cost to keep things like lead, arsenic, chlorine, and fluoride out of your lemonade!

Just Say "No" to Household Pesticides

While the risks from pesticide use are all around us, you can take one very important step to reduce your kids' exposure (and your own too) by eliminating the use of pesticides inside and outside your home. This includes pesticides applied by you and by commercial applicators. Just because a chemical is sold "over the counter" does *not* mean it's safe. And just because it's advertised as not hurting your lawn doesn't mean it won't harm you or your family or your pet. (Dursban, for instance, was one of the most widely used household pesticides in existence, until the FDA decided its use should be halted.) If annoying pest problems exist at your home, try implementing some of the methods for keeping them in check discussed in Chapter 5 that don't involve spreading toxic chemicals around your property.

Take Steps to Reduce Your Children's Exposure to
Pesticides Elsewhere

Give your children strict instructions to avoid playing on grass in the vicinity of applicators' warning flags. Check with school or day-care officials to find out if and when pesticides are being applied to facilities and classrooms, and arrange for your child to stay home on that particular day. Insist that any pesticide application at your child's school be done after the school day on Friday, and that windows be opened during the weekend to increase ventilation. Better yet, persuade school officials to eliminate toxic pesticides by introducing integrated pest-management techniques (see Chapter 5). Make your position known with teachers and administrators, and attempt to influence them and other parents to have the practice of spraying school buildings and grounds halted.

"WONDER FOODS" YOU MAY NOT HAVE HEARD ABOUT

Just as we may often be uninformed about the potential health hazards posed by certain products, so, too, are we apt to be unfamiliar with the incredible benefits that can be derived from others. Keeping our families healthy, however, calls for an awareness of both. Here, for instance, are descriptions of a couple of "wonder foods" whose protective properties most people probably still don't know about.

Coconut Oil: The "Good Fat" Finally Cleared of a Bad Rap

Could that be coconut oil included among the "healthy fats"? Surely, it must be a mistake. Isn't coconut oil considered a dietary no-no, one of those undesirable "tropical oils" that we've often been warned to avoid because of their high saturated-fat content?

Yes, there has indeed been a mistake. In essence, coconut oil has been the victim of a "bad rap," a case of mistaken identity that has succeeded in tarnishing the reputation of a valuable nutrient until quite recently.

As it turns out, the accusation made against this natural vegetable fat—that it is hazardous to heart health—was based on a faulty interpretation of animal studies done four decades ago. As Dr. Robert Atkins has noted, the studies in question utilized coconut oil that had been artificially hydrogenated, a process that created harmful trans fats, which raise blood cholesterol levels (which is why hydrogenated and partially hydrogenated foods have recently been identified as being among the real culprits in causing cardiovascular disease).

Real-life use of natural coconut oil seems to produce just the opposite results. Pacific islanders for whom it is a dietary staple have exhibited an extremely low rate of heart disease. Rather than being the health menace it was made out to be, it has been shown in studies to actually aid the recovery of heart patients, according to Mary G. Enig, Ph.D., an internationally known expert in nutrition and biochemistry and author of *Know Your Fats* (Bethesda Press, 2000).

In fact, coconut oil has been found to have another benefit that could well be lifesaving. It's a key source of lauric acid, an essential disease-fighting substance found naturally in mother's milk. Lauric acid helps protect infants against all types of pathogenic organisms. So important is lauric acid in warding off disease that it is even regarded as an important immune-system booster for people with acquired immune deficiency syndrome (AIDS).

So, yes, coconut oil is definitely back on the list of "good" oils and is today considered one of the components of a healthy diet.

Kefir: An Easy (and Tasty) Way to Bring Back the "Good Bacteria"

Children (and adults) are more susceptible to various infections and health complaints if the beneficial bacteria in their digestive tracts have been destroyed by antibiotics. Restoring a proper bacterial balance then becomes essential to make kids less prone to such problems, which include asthma, food allergies, and yeast infections. Symptoms might also include intestinal gas, bloating, cramping, and even diarrhea and constipation. What's called for in such cases is a "probiotic," which you've ingested if you've ever eaten yogurt with live cultures. The live cultures might have included *Lactobacillus acidophilus*, *Bifido bacterium*, and other species.

But one probiotic that we particularly recommend for this purpose is an ancient remedy called kefir, which contains several major strains of friendly bacteria usually not found in commercial yogurt, as well as beneficial yeasts such as *Saccharomyces kefir* and *Torula kefir*. These can help to control and eliminate destructive pathogenic yeasts in the body.[3]

In addition to restocking the digestive system with disease-fighting microbes, kefir provides a number of important nutrients, including the essential minerals calcium, magnesium, and phosphorus; tryptophan, an amino acid that combines with calcium and magnesium to help calm the nervous system; vitamins such as B_{12}, used in nerve-tissue metabolism and red blood cell formation; thiamin, which helps promote learning capacity and growth in children; and an easily absorbed complete protein containing all the essential amino acids.

Even though kefir is low in lactose and may be tolerated by many individuals with sensitivities to dairy products, if you have eliminated dairy entirely from your child's diet, you may want to try a variation called coconut water kefir. This is made by fermenting the water from young coconuts and contains no dairy. (For directions, see pages 262–265.) The recipe was conceived by nutrition expert Donna Gates, author of the best-selling *Body Ecology Diet* (B.E.D. Publications, 1996), who is one of kefir's most enthusiastic advocates.

While kefir by itself has a tangy (and quite delicious), somewhat sour taste, it is also available in a variety of flavors, such as vanilla, peach, and strawberry. A number of brands are sold in health-food stores, but the one we recommend is Helios Nutrition, since it's made with organic milk. (See "Resources" at the end of this chapter.) A number of recipes for smoothies using kefir can be found in Chapter 8.

WHEN "GOOD FOODS" MAY BE BAD FOR YOUR CHILD

There are many reasons why your child may be sensitive to certain foods. For example, some kids don't have the proper enzymes to break down a particular food, while others may produce antibodies and exhibit classic allergy symptoms, such as wheezing, hives, eye irritation, or nasal congestion. Some may be missing a mineral, enzyme, or "cofactor" needed to metabolize a food effectively, or something unique in their genetic makeup may predispose them to an intolerance. African-American kids, for example, are significantly more lactose intolerant than Caucasian children. Also, your child may not tolerate a certain food because of naturally occurring substances, such as solanine, which is found in tomatoes, potatoes, eggplants, and peppers. Wine, cheese, and sauerkraut naturally contain histamine, which can also cause adverse food reactions in susceptible individuals.

When we think of food allergies, the classic peanut or strawberry response comes to mind. These food allergies manifest themselves in obvious reactions, such as hives, swelling, and itching, and in extreme cases, life-threatening conditions such as anaphylactic shock. But adverse reactions to foods can often be very subtle and confusing to parents and even to doctors.

(If your child is lactose intolerant, see Table 3.1 for some nondairy sources of calcium.)

Causes of Food Sensitivities

Americans, especially children, eat a very repetitive diet. How many times has your toddler refused to eat anything but maca-

TABLE 3.1
Examples of Nondairy Sources of Calcium*

Food	Calcium (in milligrams)
Salmon, with bones, canned, 3 ounces	191
Collards, frozen, cooked, ½ cup	179
Dried figs, 5 pieces	135
Tofu, firm, ½ cup	118
Broccoli, fresh, cooked, ½ cup	89
Baked beans, ½ cup	80

*As a comparison, 1 cup of milk contains 300 milligrams calcium per serving.
Source: *Food: Your Miracle Medicine* by Jean Carper (New York: HarperCollins, 1993).

roni and cheese for long stretches at a time? It's this very monotonous diet that makes us more susceptible to food allergies and sensitivities. Studies have shown that 80 percent of our nutrients come from only twenty different foods; and for kids, that number is even lower. The more we eat a food over and over, the more likely we will become intolerant or sensitized to it. Even though this is not a very appetizing thought, we are ingesting pounds and pounds of food every single week, making eating one of the biggest allergenic loads our bodies have to deal with. If you include in that burden pesticides, toxic food additives, and artificial colorings and flavorings, it's amazing that your digestive tract can function at all!

Consequences of Antibiotic Abuse

Adding to the problem for children are the courses and courses of antibiotics they are given, too often for very little justifiable reason. The most common consequence of all these antibiotics is the disruption of the "friendly" bacteria in their intestines. Antibiotics kill off bacteria indiscriminately, letting the "bad," or pathogenic, bacteria take over. This causes a condition Dr. Magaziner sees frequently in children called intestinal dysbiosis. When that occurs, food cannot be processed properly and is not digested well, and that in turn makes kids susceptible to developing food sensitivities. Frequent antibiotic use can also lead to an overgrowth of intestinal yeast.

Another factor that contributes to the faulty functioning of the digestive system is anti-inflammatory drugs such as ibuprofen, aspirin, and acetaminophen. These can also lead to an imbalance of good and bad intestinal bacteria. Overuse of both prescription and over-the-counter drugs can cause a cascading effect of sometimes vague and perplexing problems such as intestinal gas, bloating, abdominal cramping, and pain.

When to Suspect That a Certain Food Might Be an Allergy Trigger

If your child has been suffering from persistent, undiagnosed medical problems or complaints such as chronic infections, headaches, runny nose, mood swings, irritability, and intestinal symptoms including bloating and gas, a thorough dietary (and environmental) evaluation is probably indicated. While the classic internist might look for conditions such as Crohn's disease, the real culprit might well be a food allergy or sensitivity that doesn't match all the conventional allergy criteria. The physician should take a thorough, detailed history, and if the child has been on several courses of antibiotics, should consider dysbiosis.

Often, you have to be a detective to uncover the real causes of a child's chronic illness, and you have to think of the most practical things to evaluate first. When the child is having allergic reactions to foods, you should consider his or her biochemistry as well. This means sometimes using nutrients and supplements to boost the child's immune system and hopefully help him or her become less susceptible. (Most children do not eat even the minimum requirements of the Recommended Dietary Allowances of the key vitamins and minerals, often necessitating the need for nutritional supplements.) The purpose is to enhance the body's ability to withstand physical "insults," whether from food, pollen, or chemicals. Just to remove a particular food may not be enough. The whole child has to be treated; you can't just say, "Don't eat apples."

The full extent of how many of today's kids are suffering from food sensitivities surprises even some experts in the field. Allan Lieberman, M.D., who specializes in environmental medicine and toxic exposures, has probably seen it all, but even he was flabbergasted to realize that a fourth of the audience of children he was addressing about allergies were experiencing daily headaches.

"Although there are many causes of headaches," Lieberman says, "my experience reveals food sensitivity to be the most common cause."

The nervous system, Lieberman points out, is "the most commonly affected organ system" showing alterations in "thinking, perception, mood, and behavior. Whether it is headaches or other nervous system signs or symptoms, food still remains the number one cause. If it is a food, it is usually the one we eat the most or crave the most."

The most frequently eaten foods, and the most frequent offenders, says Lieberman, begin with the letter C: cane, corn, cola, chocolate, citrus, cheese, chicken, and coffee. "When these foods are eliminated from our diet, many of our signs and symptoms disappear.

"The bottom line is that foods remain the number one stress to the body. No matter what chronic problems children may have or manifest, it is wise to begin looking at foods as the cause."

Often parents find that when they are attempting to remove a particular food from their child's diet, the very thing they are looking to avoid is hidden in other foods. A five-year-old is not going to sit down and eat a handful of soybeans, but soy is contained in many processed foods, not obvious unless you carefully read the labels.

Try to offer a wider variety of foods to your kids, to broaden their dietary horizon as best you can, and you'll lessen the possibility of them developing food sensitivities. Watch out for food cravings, which can indicate an allergic addiction. It's possible that an apple a day isn't the best idea after all; why not try an apple one day, a mango the next, and then a peach or a plum. (Well, you get the idea.)

Bringing Your Family on Board

Getting your kids to adapt to the kinds of lifestyle changes recommended in this book is best done by phasing such changes in gradually, by actively involving your kids in the process, and by using familiar concepts as models (for example, healthy recipes disguised as "fast foods"). Following are some practical suggestions for making healthy change a family affair.

Introducing "Picky Eaters" to a Variety of Healthier Foods

You probably remember them from your own childhood: the customary admonitions about eating that included, "Don't spoil your appetite for dinner" and "Be sure and clean your plate." But if you really want your kids to be receptive to a healthier diet, it might well be time to dispense with such conventional wisdom and adopt a more flexible and imaginative approach, one that incorporates the following recommendations.

Don't Worry About Them "Spoiling Their Appetite"

Little kids have little tummies that can't necessarily accommodate what you might consider a "regular" portion of food. Rather than eating full-course meals, it is often better for them to have healthy snacks throughout the day, maybe every three to four hours. The same applies to older kids. Having sliced fruit, crackers, raw veggies, and cheese available is an excellent way to keep up with their nutritional needs. What's important is making sure they get the proper foods during the course of a day, not monitoring portion size or insisting that they eat everything they're given for breakfast, lunch, and dinner.

Show the "Clean Plate" the Gate

Not only does the battle over having a clean plate make dinner a miserable experience, but studies have shown that children who are overfed are much more likely to be obese as adults. Hold on—overfed, you say? My toddler eats only two bites for lunch and one for dinner, so how can I be overfeeding him even if I get him to clean his plate? The late pediatrician Dr. Robert S. Mendelsohn, noted in his book *How to Raise a Healthy Child . . . in Spite of Your Doctor* (Ballantine Books, 1987) that a child's appetite varies from day to day and year to year for many reasons: "The child, whether he is a baby or in his teens, will eat what he needs. No child, unless he or she is suffering from anorexia nervosa, will ever starve to death if food is available."

Get Kids Involved in Food Preparation

If you ever had an Easy Bake Oven as a kid, you know that no matter how silly, messy, or even vile tasting your creation was, you and your fellow bakers consumed it eagerly. The same rule applies where real food is concerned. Depending on their age, kids can participate in some part of food preparation, be it measuring, mixing, peeling, slicing, or even helping decide what to make for lunch or dinner. Such active participation, you'll discover, will generally extend to the eating part as well. We also suggest that you periodically take your children food shopping with you, especially to a health-food store, so they can participate in food selection. The earlier they start making healthy choices on their own, the better.

Don't Overwhelm Kids with New Foods

Think of yourself as an explorer in a strange land. People are constantly presenting you with things to eat—funny-looking things they keep reassuring you are delicious and good for you. You probably would be longing for the familiar comforts of home and a peanut butter and jelly sandwich. One of the best and hardest parts of being a kid is the combination of wonder and apprehension that surrounds new things. So when you introduce picky eaters to a new "healthy" food, don't make a big deal out of it. Integrate the new food with the familiar standbys like whole-grain macaroni and cheese (and preferably not the canned or frozen varieties, which are laced with additives), and give them an opportunity to "discover" the new food for themselves. You may be pleasantly surprised when they actually ask for it on their own.

Encourage Them to Take "Just One Bite"

A whole plate of anything can be very intimidating. Why not try the "just one bite" approach? You'll be surprised at a kid's willingness to take one bite of practically anything, no matter how unfamiliar or unappetizing it might seem. And who knows? That one bite may very well lead to another. Also, keep in mind that you, as a parent, need to set an example and show your child that you enjoy the food as well. If you or your spouse complain about a particular food, chances are your child will also dislike that food.

Don't Bribe or Describe

Eating is not a contest with a potential reward at the end. Don't make a bowl of ice cream the prize for eating spinach, as if the spinach is something unpleasant. Also, kids don't need descriptions of the new foods you may be serving. You're not a waiter or waitress reciting the specials of the day. Put it on the table and see what happens.

FAKE FOOD CITATION
Green Ketchup and Blue Fries

As food companies have shown, there are all kinds of imaginative ways of turning breakfast food into "kid stuff," but what about items more commonly associated with lunch and dinner—like ketchup, for example? Now that's a condiment of a different color—green, to be precise.

If the product's appearance seems unnatural, that's exactly what it is. No, it's not made from green tomatoes; two artificial colors do the trick—Yellow Number 5 and Blue Number 1 Aluminum Lake. That last one, incidentally, contains actual aluminum in the form of aluminum hydroxide, and while the FDA claims it's perfectly safe, some health experts have urged that ingestion of aluminum be avoided because it has been found in the brains of Alzheimer's patients. Avoiding such synthetic dyes whenever possible, of course, is one of the things you need to do in making your kids chemical-free.

Now, as the perfect partner to green ketchup, come blue French fries.

In an editorial from *Just-Food.com*, a food industry Web site, managing editor Catherine Sleep comments: "I agree it's not the job of manufacturers to teach our children to eat well, that's the job of parents. But do they have to make it so hard? How about a little more investment in making genuinely healthful food appeal to kids? Now that would really be something to be proud of." Sleep adds, "Let's try to love the food around us without distorting it past the point of recognition."

Serve Raw Vegetables Instead of Cooked Ones

Often, raw veggies have much more appeal to kids than cooked ones. For one thing, they're finger foods and seem much friend-lier. Then again, they can be dipped in salsa and bean- or yogurt-based dressings, which even picky eaters are more prone to like.

Mix Veggies into Other Food Dishes

Carrots, red peppers, cucumbers, and zucchini, to name a few, can easily be shredded or grated and added to numerous main and side dishes without suspicion from a vegetable-phobic kid. Don't forget about homemade zucchini and carrot breads. Although fresh is best, it's better they eat their veggies in some form rather than not at all.

Don't Let Them Fill Up on Liquids

Again, kids don't have that much room in their stomachs. Certainly, they need fluids, but constant slurping from little juice boxes is certain to discourage them from wanting to participate in dinner. While juices can provide some nutrition (they usually have added vitamin C), they don't take the place of actual food.

Don't Be Overly Concerned with Food Obsessions

Kids often favor certain foods and snub others, but that need not be a cause of consternation. As Dr. Mendelsohn points out, "Kids don't have to eat everything. As long as he is getting a basic diet, with all of the food groups represented, it isn't imperative that he eat every vegetable." Rather than worrying about a kid who seems to consume large quantities of a certain food (we're talking about things like bananas and apples here, not Twinkies), your concern would be better directed at making sure you serve the organic version of the favorite food of the week. Certainly, having a totally organic diet would be best, but if that's not feasible, you should definitely buy the organic version of any food that you and your kids eat the most to prevent consuming higher amounts of any particular type of pesticide.

What Kids Should Ideally Be Eating

As you phase in changes in your family's daily diet, you might want to keep in mind the long-term objective of gradually converting your kids to one that's completely natural and chemical-free. Here's a summary of what they should ideally be eating.

FAKE FOOD CITATION
Fruit Beverages

What is a fruit beverage anyway? One thing is for sure: It's definitely not fruit juice (or frequently, up to 95 percent of its contents aren't).

Consumer perception of just what some of these products are supposed to be has played a big part in their success. One, an orange-juicelike liquid that requires no refrigeration prior to opening (not being fresh juice) is typically found in the perishable drink section, side by side with the real orange juice. This tactic has not gone unnoticed by marketing specialists. "It is possible . . . that this positioning has caused certain consumers to associate this product with the same health benefits as pure fruit juices in spite of its relatively low juice content," states one industry report.[4]

Even though an eight-ounce serving typically will provide 100 percent of the government-recommended allowance for vitamin C, your kids may also get high-fructose corn syrup, modified food starch, cottonseed oil, gellan gum, guar gum, cellulose gum, xanthan gum, two preservatives, and Yellow Numbers 5 and 6.

If it's orange juice you want, there are plenty of ready-made brands from which to choose that contain no added water, sugar, or colorings. Or better yet, why not buy some oranges, slice them in half, and squeeze them? With an electric juice squeezer, it takes only a few minutes—less time than it takes to read the labels and try to figure out what these fruit beverages really are.

Organic Fresh Fruits and Vegetables

How about orange or apple slices instead of chips as a snack? Many kids also enjoy grapes, peaches, pears, kiwis, strawberries, blueberries, pineapple, nectarines, melon, and bananas. Or how about baby carrots or cucumber slices? Dr. Magaziner's kids snack on slices of red, yellow, and orange peppers; grape tomatoes; broccoli; mushrooms; and snap peas. Give these a try. You may be surprised at how much your child enjoys them, especially when combined with a healthy dip.

NONDAIRY BEVERAGES AND DESSERTS

If your child is lactose intolerant, you can still give him or her healthy drinks that are milklike in consistency and desserts that are cool and creamy like ice cream. Following are some popular examples. Note, however, that some of the desserts may contain a fair amount of sugar.

- Rice beverages, such as Rice Dream brand, which comes in plain, carob, and vanilla flavors
- Soy beverages, such as White Wave Silk brand, which comes in plain, vanilla, chocolate, egg nog, and chai flavors; Edensoy brand, which comes in plain, carob, and vanilla flavors; Westbrae brand, which comes in plain and vanilla flavors; as well as Hansen's Natural Soy Smoothie brand, which comes in a variety of fruit flavors
- Almond beverages, such as Pacific and Blue Diamond brands, which come in plain, vanilla, and chocolate flavors; and Amazake brand, which comes in almond flavor
- Sorbet, which comes in all the standard flavors, including vanilla, chocolate, and fruit flavors
- Rice- and almond-beverage-based frozen desserts, which come in the standard flavors

Organic Whole-Grain Cereals and Crackers

Organic cereals containing rice, wheat, oats, corn, or kamut can also double as snack foods. Such products, which are now carried by many supermarkets, do not contain white sugar and are apt to be high in beneficial fiber, vitamins, minerals, and antioxidants. Organic graham crackers and animal crackers are also widely available.

Organic Air-Popped Popcorn and Dried Fruits

Within five minutes you can make organic air-popped popcorn with an air popper. You can also make your own trail mix with dried fruits and nuts. Dried fruits are extremely sweet and should satisfy the sweet tooth of even a confirmed sugar addict.

Organic Dairy Products and Eggs

Buying dairy products made with organic milk is the only real assurance you have that the milk they contain did not come from cows treated with bovine growth hormone (BGH). BGH-treated cows are more prone to infections and therefore receive more antibiotics, which are passed along with their milk. Also, no one really knows the risks involved in consuming milk and milk products from BGH-treated cows, which some evidence suggests may increase the chances of developing breast and prostate cancer.

Dr. Enig is among the nutrition experts who recommend that children eat at least an egg a day. Conventional eggs, however, come from chickens that were given antibiotics and were exposed to pesticides and other chemicals in their food and water. Organic eggs are raised without growth hormones, antibiotics, and pesticides, and are readily available in health-food stores and some supermarkets. Frequent ingestion of antibiotic-laden food can increase your child's risk of antibiotic resistance and yeast infections.

Organic Meats and Poultry

Again, most conventionally raised farm animals are permanently confined, sprayed with pesticides, shot up with antibiotics, and given feed containing more chemicals. Antibiotic resistance in people caused by ingesting these drugs from animal sources is a very real threat. If you expect antibiotics to work when you need them, you can't be exposed to them constantly, which makes organic meat and poultry the best choice for nonvegetarians.

Fish and Other Foods Containing "Good Fats"

Perhaps reacting to the news that nearly 60 percent of adults and 30 percent of kids in the United States are now considered overweight, and that obesity is a cause of illness and death, many of us have gone overboard in our quest to eliminate fat from our diet. What we need to remember, however, is that children need appropriate, *good-quality* dietary fats and cannot develop properly without them, as they are necessary sources of vitamins A and D and ensure the proper absorption of vitamin B_{12}.

According to Dr. Enig, the amount of fats a child requires on a daily basis is approximately 50 to 55 percent of the total calories consumed for children up to two years of age, 45 percent of total caloric intake at age six, and 40 percent at age ten, gradually decreasing to 30 percent by age eighteen.

In contrast to the assumption of recent years that all fat is unhealthy, what we now know is that the idea of throwing all fat into a single vat is dangerous oversimplification. Fats, like foods themselves, may be good or bad for us depending on their chemical makeup and nutritional value. And by avoiding anything labeled "fat," we deprive our bodies of certain essential nutrients and cushions that nature intended to help support various functions and protect us from disease.

Dr. Enig is among the nutritional experts who advocate consumption of the omega-3 fatty acids, found in both flaxseed oil and various types of fish. As noted earlier in this chapter, she's also an advocate of coconut oil and recommends products made from desiccated or whole coconuts, such as macaroons and coconut milk, for their lauric acid content. (Small amounts of lauric acid are present in full-fat dairy products.)

For many of us, the word "cholesterol" has likewise come to represent a threat to our health. But cholesterol, as Dr. Enig points out, is the body's repair substance, one needed for proper brain function and hormonal balance.

When using fats and oils, however. Dr. Enig cautions against consuming any one exclusively, since different fats and oils contain the different fatty acids needed by the body. She also warns consumers to throw away any fats and oils that have become rancid, even if they were expensive.

Your Favorite Food Could Just Be the Perfect Food

Let's see: It's got bread, vegetables, and dairy; possibly some meat; not to mention fat; and if you live in California, probably some fruit, too. Shouldn't that make pizza a perfect food, an ideal combination of the essential elements that make up the "new" food pyramid?

While it might sound like you've got all the bases covered when it comes to adequate nutrition, the trouble with pizza is about the same as the trouble with the notorious food pyramid itself. The food pyramid is the nutritional edifice constructed on the site of what was originally known as the "four food groups" (meat, dairy, produce, and grains) in 1992 when the U.S. government revised its orientation of what it considers a balanced diet.

The problems with the food pyramid are that:

- It makes no distinction between hydrogenated oils, or animal fats, and the more healthful fats from plants and vegetable sources.
- It makes no distinction between whole grains and white flour.
- It makes no distinction between fresh fruits and vegetables and canned ones that have had their nutrients cooked out.[5]

The ingredients in pizza, unfortunately, all too often tend to be of the hydrogenated, white, and canned variety. That's not to say, however, that pizza can't be a source of truly good and diverse nutrition. Pizza, fortunately, does contain tomatoes, which are rich in the phytonutrient lycopene, associated with lowering the risk for heart disease, prostate cancer, and more recently, osteoporosis.

Just as you can have your own personalized food pyramid,

consisting of good fats, whole grains, and fresh, organic vegetables, you can also improve your pizza. Instead of a typical "white bread" pizza, why not make one out of whole-grain flour, organic tomatoes and cheese, and high-quality olive oil, then top it off with fresh, organic vegetables and perhaps some artichoke hearts? Made the right way, pizza can be as healthy an eating experience for your family as it is enjoyable.

SHOULD KIDS TAKE NUTRITIONAL SUPPLEMENTS?

In an ideal world, we would all eat six or more servings of fruits and vegetables a day. We would consume this colorful bounty all gathered around the dinner table, sharing stories and having meaningful conversations about school, work, and important events. Do we hear you laughing?

Hopefully, what you've read in this book so far has encouraged you to include more healthful foods in your kids' diet, which is the best way to provide them with vitamins, minerals, and other nutrients. But even if your breakfasts, lunches, and dinners are on the right nutritional track, it's still a good idea to include certain supplements for kids, even ones as young as two. In some cases, they can even help kids to detoxify.

A Multivitamin a Day Can Keep Infections at Bay

Since kids generally don't eat the minimum requirements of fruits and vegetables every day, they are usually deficient in trace minerals and antioxidants. That's why Dr. Magaziner and other experts recommend a multivitamin-and-mineral supplement every day, but not just any such supplement. Make sure the one you choose doesn't contain aspartame or artificial colors or flavorings, as many do. You can buy children's multivitamin-and-mineral supplements in chewable, liquid, and powder forms.

Children's multivitamin-and-mineral supplements characteristically include very small amounts of vitamins B, C, and E, as well as of folic acid and trace minerals such as calcium, magnesium, and zinc. Therefore, if your child has recurrent infections or colds, some extra vitamin C is also a good idea. For children under the age of ten, 250 milligrams of extra C can be helpful to boost the immune system; for older kids, you can go up to 1,000 milligrams a day. This added protection is especially important when school starts in the fall, and can be continued throughout the winter season.

Supplement Solutions for "Special Problems"

In addition to a good multivitamin-and-mineral supplement, there are supplements specifically for kids who need some extra help. Children who have autism or autism-like tendencies, ADD, recurrent infections, and/or difficulty concentrating or sleeping, to name just a few problems, can benefit from taking some of the supplements listed below.

Calcium and Magnesium

As good team players, calcium and magnesium work together in the body and should therefore be taken together. (You can easily find them combined.) Dr. Magaziner likes a two-to-one ratio: two parts calcium to one part magnesium. This supplement is an excellent addition for children on a dairy-free diet, as well as for those who get frequent colds or infections, are hyperactive, or show autistic tendencies or developmental delays.

Most kids and adults do not get enough magnesium. Furthermore, the more stress we're under, the more magnesium we lose and, therefore, the more we need. Magnesium has been shown to have a calming effect and to help with muscle spasms and leg cramps.

A supplement of about 500 milligrams of calcium and 250 milligrams of magnesium should be sufficient. But a note of caution: Avoid oyster shell calcium supplements, as they are the most likely to still contain lead. Calcium citrate is a recommended form.

DHA and Essential Fatty Acids

Docosahexaenoic acid (DHA), a very safe supplement derived from fish, can help kids who have vision or learning problems, as well as those suffering from eczema. (Vitamin C and zinc are recommended for eczema as well.) Because DHA occurs naturally in breast milk, infants fed exclusively on formula are more susceptible to a DHA deficiency.

Flaxseed, like DHA, is high in the omega-3 fatty acids and useful for improving awareness and helping constipation. Flaxseed can be taken as a powder, in doses of one-half to one teaspoon a day, added to breakfast cereals or smoothies (a kefir smoothie is an excellent idea). Flaxseed oil can be used at the same dosage, also added to smoothies or incorporated into oatmeal or other cooked cereals *after* cooking. (Do not cook with flaxseed oil, as heat destroys its beneficial properties.) Also, flaxseed oil should be kept in the refrigerator. DHA is not very tasty, but you should be able to find a flavored DHA supplement without much trouble.

Primrose oil contains omega-6 fatty acids and is excellent for detoxification, as well as for helping psoriasis and eczema. Certain drugs, such as steroids taken for asthma, can have an adverse effect on the liver and slow down its ability to detoxify the body. Primrose oil can help counteract that effect. Dr. Magaziner recommends 500 milligrams a day for kids under the age of ten and up to 1,300 milligrams a day for older ones. Vitamin C is also useful in the detoxifying process.

Probiotics

As discussed earlier in this Chapter, probiotics are naturally occurring "friendly" bacteria that need to be replaced in children who have taken a course of antibiotics. Supplements of acidophilus or bifidus may be needed not only if kids have taken antibiotics, but also if they have a lot of mucus and congestion. In addition, these probiotics are good for children suffering from rectal itching and intestinal pain. Kefir is a probiotic and an excellent way to repopulate the good bacteria in the intestinal tract. However, for kids on a dairy-free diet, it's best to go with probiotic supplements or coconut water kefir (see pages 262–265). Store acidophilus and bifidus supplements in the refrigerator.

Zinc

Zinc has been shown to improve focus and concentration, alleviate eczema, stimulate the appetite, boost the immune system, and help with learning disabilities.

We're not talking about those zinc lozenges that you take several times a day at the onset of a cold and that have about 23 milligrams per pill (too much to take on an ongoing basis). What we're talking about is a zinc supplement of about 15 milligrams a day.

Zinc is a crucial mineral of which most of us who eat a refined diet don't get enough. (White spots on the fingernails are a definite sign of a zinc deficiency.) A course of zinc supplements to correct an imbalance should run about six months.

As an ancient proverb notes, "A journey of a thousand miles begins with a single step." By taking any one of the steps recommended in this chapter, you'll begin leading your kids on one of the most important journeys of their lives—a trek out of the largely invisible toxic rut in which the majority of people in our chemical-drenched society are stuck. All you need do is get them far enough along the road, and you'll be delighted to find them proceeding all on their own.

RESOURCES

General Health

The Body Ecology Diet
Web site: www.bodyecologydiet.com
    Information and advice from Donna Gates, author of the best-selling *Body Ecology Diet* (B.E.D. Publications, 1996), for people suffering from candidiasis and other conditions.

The Magaziner Center for Wellness and Anti-Aging Medicine
Web site: www.drmagaziner.com
    Information on foods, supplements, and alternative treatment options for various health problems and conditions.

Kefir

Helios Nutrition
Web site: www.heliosnutrition.com
    Information about Helios Nutrition organic kefir with FOS.

Kefir: The Ancient Antidote for Modern Maladies
Web site: www.kefir.net
    Nutritional facts and recipes about kefir.

Supplements

iVillage Market
Web site: http://shop.ivillage.com/
    The online women's home, health, family, and career network. Offers iVillage Solutions brand of chewable multivitamin-and-mineral supplement called Mighty Multis for Kids, as well as Mighty C for Kids. Mighty Multis for Kids provides twenty-three essential vitamins and minerals derived from natural plant sources with no synthetic chemicals. Mighty C for Kids is a natural, chewable vitamin C. Products are available online.

Nature's Plus
548 Broadhollow Road
Melville, NY 11747
Telephone: 800-937-0500
E-mail: info@naturesplus.com
Web site: www.naturesplus.com
   Offers Animal Parade line of natural supplements for infants
and children. Products available in health-food stores.

Nutrition Now
6350 Northeast Campus Drive
Vancouver, WA 98661
E-mail: nnow@nutritionnow.com
Web site: www.nutritionnow.com
   Offers Rhino line of natural supplements, including calcium,
FOS, and acidophilus. Products are available in health-food
stores.

PART TWO

A CHEMICAL-FREE HOME ZONE AND ENVIRONMENT

❋ 4 ❋

Setting Aside Pesticides

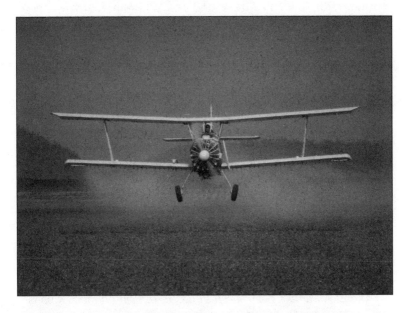

*"Pesticide use is an unnecessary, life-destroying activity.
Risk assessment arranges deck chairs on the* Titanic. *Let's
refuse to get on board."*
>   —Mary O'Brien, staff scientist, Environmental
>   Research Foundation

*By their very nature, most pesticides create some risk of
harm to humans, animals, or the environment because they
are designed to kill or otherwise adversely affect living
organisms.*
>   —United States Environmental Protection Agency

What You'll Find in This Chapter

Pesticides poison more than bugs. In the United States, 1.2 billion pounds of these chemicals are used each year (three-fourths in farming). With this dependency on quick, toxic fixes, it's certainly no surprise we are killing fish, birds, and beneficial insects, and poisoning our food, soil, water, and air, along with our farm workers, our kids, and ourselves.

Schools may be ignorant of toxic hazards. That's why it's so important for you to learn what kinds of poisons your child's school may be using and to try to educate the educators about the dangers of exposing kids to pesticides that can both make them sick and interfere with their ability to learn.

Beware of tents and tarps. Tented houses (structures that have been temporarily sealed in plastic enclosures that resemble circus tents) and tarped fields are indicators of structural or soil fumigation with a chemical called methyl bromide, an extremely lethal poison capable of killing any living thing it encounters, including you and the members of your family. The facts that methyl bromide has claimed victims of all ages and is now believed to pose a powerful threat to the earth's protective ozone layer, however, so far haven't been sufficient to get it removed from the market—not with influential agribusiness interests supporting legislators who have found ways to keep it in circulation. Which means it's up to you to make sure your children aren't exposed to this toxic serial killer.

The EPA permits pesticide residues to remain on food. It uses measurements called "tolerances," the maximum legal amounts allowed in the food you eat. Your fruit salad, for instance, could have multiple traces of pesticides in it, all quite legal, from a variety of chemicals applied to different fruits. The Food Quality Protection Act was supposed to require that tolerances be set more stringently than before, with a tenfold safety factor if necessary, to protect kids if there were "data gaps" on how certain chemicals might affect developing brains and nervous systems. But so far, it's been done in only a fraction of cases.

Things You Can Do Now!

- You don't have to wait for the EPA to set safer standards for you and your kids. Set your own standards by using certified organic foods whenever possible or at least for the foods you and your kids eat the most.

- Find out if and when your kids' school or day-care facility will be treated with chemicals and discuss the alternatives. Be on the lookout for brown or wilting weeds, a definite tip-off that pesticides have been sprayed.
- Instruct your kids to keep off the grass whenever they see those warning flags on a lawn.
- Don't use flea collars on your pets.
- Take your shoes off at the door. Chemicals can be tracked in from the outside and picked up by crawling toddlers and kids playing on the floor.
- If you use well water, have it tested for pesticide contamination and toxic metals such as lead.

What we commonly call "pests" have been around a lot longer than people have. And there are times when they constitute a real nuisance—when they transmit disease, for instance, or decimate crops. Most of the time, however, bugs, weeds, and vermin are simply annoying, irritating, or inconvenient. But to the makers and promoters of pesticides, any intrusion on residential or agricultural property by life-forms deemed "undesirable" is reason enough for us to unleash a torrent of toxic chemicals on the landscape, if not inside our very homes. And as such poisons continue to accumulate in our environment and our bodies, increasing the likelihood that we—and especially our children—will develop cancer or some serious neurodegenerative affliction, it might seem like we've substituted a far worse problem for the one we're trying to eliminate. But as has become more and more apparent, in the long run all that those poisonous sprays have managed to do is to make the pests they were meant to eliminate impervious to their effects, even as we suffer the consequences.

THE PESTICIDE PENALTY

In the year 2000, the EPA finally got around to taking a second look at one of the most commonly used insecticides on the market and didn't like what it saw. As a result, the agency ordered the chemical chlorpyrifos, more commonly known by the brand names Dursban and Lorsban, phased out for nearly all indoor and outdoor residential uses. It also halted its use, as of the end of 2001, in schools, parks, and other settings where children might be exposed, and ordered certain agricultural uses of the chemical reduced.

While certainly welcome news to environmental organizations and parents, the action was also bad news to the public in the sense that it reflected just how misplaced our confidence actually has been in the supposed "safety" of federally registered pesticides. No more could we take for granted the idea that if the government allows it, it must be okay.

"Through this review, EPA has determined that chlorpyrifos, as currently used, does not provide an adequate margin of protection for children," notes an EPA Web site on the subject. "This action adds a greater measure of protection for children by reducing/eliminating the most important sources of exposure."[1] But while attempting to allay public concern about the significance of such exposure, the EPA can't conceal the fact that chlorpyrifos has been routinely used for years (and can still be used until supplies run out) in many of the places where children are most apt to come into contact with it, including classrooms, school cafeterias, and lockers.

What kind of damage might such exposure produce? To quote a Cornell University fact sheet on chlorpyrifos issued in 1999, "There is clear evidence that it is toxic to the nervous system. Hence, unnecessary exposure to this chemical and exposure to children, especially toddlers, should be minimized."[2] That's not surprising, however, when one considers that it's one of a class of pesticides, called organophosphates, that are deliberately intended to poison the nervous systems of pests by interfering with an enzyme in the brain called acetylchlolinesterase. According to the Center for Children's Health and the Environment of the Mount Sinai School of Medicine, "There is substantial evidence from animal studies that chronic, low-level exposure to organo-

phosphates affects neurodevelopment and neurobehavioral functioning in developing animals," and that it can affect children's
developing nervous systems in a similar manner. The results, the
center notes, may include "lower cognitive function, behavior
disorders, and other subtle neurological deficits." Research findings also suggest that organophosphates disrupt the autonomic
nervous system, which controls the motor functioning of the lungs,
and "may be among the preventable causes of childhood asthma."[3]

A "Textbook Case" of What Pesticide Exposure Can Do

Dr. Allan Lieberman, a specialist in occupational and environmental medicine in Charleston, South Carolina, has seen firsthand the results of organophosphate exposure in children. One
of his patients, "C.C.," was exposed to an organophosphate chemical while his school was being treated for termites. The pesticide,
instead of going into the ground, was injected from an outside
wall into the classroom; C.C. and his classmates used paper towels to wipe up the mysterious liquid.

C.C. began to suffer headaches, fatigue, spaciness, and a dramatic loss in memory. Once a superior student, the teenager now
was experiencing a significant decline in visual, cognitive, perceptual, and memory functions.

Based on what "most physicians are taught about organophosphate pesticide poisoning, it was difficult to believe that this student
could have been injured from this exposure," comments Dr. Lieberman. "However, this is exactly what happened. Organophosphate
pesticide poisoning is more pervasive than realized. It is the most
commonly used [type of] home and garden pesticide and there is
almost nowhere anyone can go that they are not exposed. This
student had chronic organophosphate pesticide–induced neu-
ropsychiatric disorder (COPIND). It can occur years after the initial exposure or from chronic low-level exposure which is so low
you don't even know you have been exposed. This is contrary to
established principles of toxicology, where dose determines toxic-

ity. Once a person has been initially exposed, they may react to very low levels subsequently.

"Pesticides in general and organophosphate pesticides in particular," adds Dr. Lieberman, "should not be used in a home." Three years after his initial exposure to the pesticide (during which he underwent an intense program of biodetoxification the first four weeks, followed by an ongoing maintenance program), C.C.'s concentration has improved; however, he is extremely chemically sensitive. Exposure to odors and chemicals still causes brain fog and a loss in concentration.

Could the dramatic rises in both attention deficit disorder and asthma rates among school children be part of the penalty we're now paying for the proliferation of pesticides in our everyday environment? The companies that manufacture these products would have you believe that whatever risks their use involves are far outweighed by their supposed benefits. But it's become more and more evident that the practice of pouring multiple poisons into our environment has ended up perpetuating the very problems it's supposed to solve. It has also created a whole slew of new ones, and we may not yet have even become fully aware of some of them.

Take the current rise in cases of childhood asthma, for instance. To hear the manufacturers of organophosphate insecticides tell it, such products help to control cockroaches, which may trigger asthmatic reactions in children. What they fail to mention is that the sprays themselves may be doing more harm than good in this respect, and that far less toxic and less allergy-inducing control methods are readily available.

The biggest argument made by the pesticide industry, of course, is that its products help stave off mass famine by eliminating insects and weeds, which reduce the sizes of crop yields. This completely ignores what environmentalists have repeatedly stressed and experience has consistently proven—that toxic chemicals are at best a "quick fix" that fails to address the root causes of the problem. Then, too, repeated exposures often cause pests to become immune to their effects, resulting in a vicious cycle of ever more powerful poisons having to be used to control them. "Pesticides kill or damage pests, sometimes very effectively," notes the Northwest Coalition for Alternatives to Pesticides (NCAP). But "what they don't do, is solve pest problems," as evidenced by "an estimated 4.4 billion applications . . . made annually in homes, yards and gardens."[4]

This vicious cycle of pesticide amplification goes back to the early 1940s when dichlorodiphenyltrichloroethane (DDT) was first being promoted as a magic bullet. Hailed as the "wonder chemical" by the U.S. Army, DDT initially worked so well at stopping outbreaks of serious diseases such as malaria that the Swiss chemist who discovered it in 1939, Paul Herman Mueller, won a Nobel Prize for physiology and medicine. This incredible killing ability didn't go unnoticed by agricultural scientists. Dramatic increases in crop yields using DDT and other synthetic insecticides so excited entomologists of the day that they believed their use could bring about the elimination of pests, rather than simply control of them.[5]

But organochlorine chemicals such as DDT, which are actually nerve poisons (and the predecessors to organophosphates), turned out to have disastrous side effects, and their use had unintended consequences. Not only do they remain in the environment for long periods of time (it takes three to ten years for 50 percent of DDT to break down in soil), but they dissolve and store easily in fat, and actually move up the food chain, becoming more concentrated as they go, in a process called biomagnification. In 1954, western grebes, birds that frequented Clear Lake, California, began dying in large numbers. The lake, which had been treated with a relative of DDT in 1949 for gnats, had levels of the chemical 100,000 times lower than did the birds. The insecticide had concentrated as it moved up the food chain, from the plankton in the lake to the fish that ate the plankton, to the fish-eating fish, to the grebes that ate the fish.[6]

In much the same way, these chemicals are found in the fatty tissue and breast milk of people everywhere in the world, even in Eskimos living in the Arctic Circle, where they have never been used.[7] We're exposed through our daily diet of meat, dairy, fish, fruit, and vegetables, which are all affected by the bioaccumulation of these chemicals that were going to save the world. In 1972, the widespread toxic effects of DDT led to its becoming the very first synthetic pesticide to be banned in the United States. The power of these bug killers seemed miraculous, too good to be true, and it was. In a bizarre turn, it became apparent that the ever-increasing use of these chemicals was creating new pest problems—resurgence and resistance. As early as the 1940s, it was discovered that chemicals such as DDT caused giant outbreaks of the very pests they were meant to control by destroying their natural predators. (One study found the insect levels more than 1,250 times higher on DDT-sprayed trees than on unsprayed ones.) Not only was it found that the original pest could resurge at higher levels after pesticide use, but in an even more unique phenomenon, insects that originally were not a problem suddenly multiplied to "pest" level after chemical treatment[8] (that is, they began to appear in large numbers).

By contrast, organic agriculture (discussed in Chapter 7) offers more lasting solutions to pest problems with none of the penalties we are now paying for the use of poisonous pesticides, penalties that include:

- Learning disabilities and behavioral problems in children
- Adverse health effects in adults ranging from headaches and memory problems to life-altering multiple chemical sensitivity
- Increased risks of cancer and neurological illnesses such as Parkinson's disease, which have been increasingly linked to pesticide exposure
- An estimated 20,000 deaths from pesticide poisonings per year on a worldwide basis
- Approximately 67,000 annual cases of accidental nonfatal pesticide poisoning in the United States per year
- Between 10,000 and 20,000 cases of physician-diagnosed, pesticide-related illnesses and injuries per year among farm

workers alone in the United States, with many more going unreported (since no comprehensive national data now exist)[9]

- An estimated 67 million annual bird deaths[10] and 6 to 14 million fish deaths from pesticide exposure in the United States
- Substantial damage to honeybees and other beneficial insects
- Contamination of drinking water, as evidenced by the discovery of weed killer in the tap water of twenty-eight out of twenty-nine cities tested in the Midwest[11]
- Biomagnification of pesticides and further amplification of the amount of poison as it moves up the food chain
- Ill effects suffered by people living downwind of fields and lawns that have been sprayed or fumigated as a result of pesticide drift
- Increases in asthma and respiratory infections

"Do You Know What Your Children Are Being Exposed to at School?"

In the fall of 2000, Dr. Lieberman treated a nine-year-old boy, "C.F.," who developed chronic outbreaks of hives, along with anxious behavior, excessive crying, nausea, vomiting, congestion, and sinusitis soon after returning to school from summer vacation.

At first, the school identified what appeared to be multiple insect bites on C.F.'s skin and on that of other classmates as being caused by sand fleas, and sprayed the classroom with a synthetic pyrethroid pesticide. After a second round of pesticides was used, the children in the classroom experienced episodes of nausea and vomiting. Still, more pesticides were applied. By now, more children, as well as the teacher, were developing skin problems.

The state division of environmental control came to investigate, concluding that the problems were psychosomatic. Despite the state's diagnosis, and despite a thorough cleaning of the classrooms during the Christmas break, the children broke out with hivelike lesions and swelling as soon as they returned to school.

When C.F. returned to the classroom, he didn't even have to go inside to get a reaction; just standing in the doorway was enough. Dr. Lieberman had him placed in a biodetoxification program for a week, with sauna therapy and lymphatic massage, which seemed to bring out a strong chemical odor in the child.

"This is a fascinating case," says Dr. Lieberman, "as it raises the question: 'Do you know what your children are being exposed to at school?' When I investigated this case, I found out that prior to the school opening, it had been treated with an organophosphate pesticide. Within four days of opening, the whole school was again sprayed with a synthetic pyrethroid and then six more times over the next two months."

Although it is possible that the sand fleas had some role in the outbreak, the massive spraying of the pesticides was a much greater cause of injury, according to Dr. Lieberman. "Skin lesions are a common manifestation of pyrethroid pesticide exposure. Symptoms of fatigue, irritability to outright aggressiveness along with depression and affective disorders are associated with organophosphate pesticide exposure," as are changes in visual-motor skills and (especially) handwriting, as demonstrated in a study done on pesticide exposure in Mexico.

"I see only a few children brought [into the office] because of injuries suffered from pesticide exposure in contrast to seeing many teachers," says Dr. Lieberman. But that's because "children are so often sick that illnesses are not associated with possible pesticide exposure, whereas teachers seem more aware of adverse environmental triggers. Parents should demand—by legislation if necessary—that no toxic chemicals, including pesticides, be used in schools," he adds.

Saner Solutions for Schools

It was a chance event eight years ago that brought Stephen Tvedten and Bob McClintock together, sort of a chemical connection. McClintock, assistant superintendent of business for the Northmont School District near Dayton, Ohio, first heard of Tvedten through a parent whose home had been rendered uninhabitable by a termite treatment.

"This family had to move out of their house; they basically boarded it up and left," says McClintock.

Although the family left their contaminated home behind, the results lingered. Sensitized to chemicals, they could no longer tolerate further exposures, and while searching for help, they found Tvedten.

" 'I got the kids out of the house, but you use pesticides in school, don't you?' " McClintock recalled the father asking him. "I told him, 'Yes, we do,' and he said, 'Let me introduce you to Stephen Tvedten.' "

A man on a mission, Tvedten made the six-hour trip from Michigan after McClintock agreed to a meeting. "I had to show I could remove the pests inside and outside," says Tvedten. And that he has since accomplished without using any chemical pesticides.

"Some of the methods Steve uses are many of the things that our parents and grandparents did," says McClintock. "His program has been excellent in making people more aware that we can do these things naturally."

When he first arrived at Northmont, Tvedten attended a meeting at which several conventional pest-control-firm representatives were present. They referred to his methods as "voodoo pest control," he recalls. But he was determined to prove otherwise, and not just "one school at a time," as was suggested to him. "How would you explain to a mother that one child is going to a school that uses alternatives, and one is going to a school that uses pesticides?"

Tvedten's approach prevailed, and he was charged with solving the pest problems of the entire district, which includes seven elementary schools, a middle school, and a high school, accommodating approximately 5,800 students in all. Eight years later, he was still serving as the district's consultant, keeping the schools free of both pests and pesticides, and providing training to the custodial staff in chemical-free pest management.

McClintock, for one, has been impressed with the results. "Do research, find out what's available in your area," is his advice to other school districts. "There are good alternatives."

Bringing the Lesson Home

As a parent, how do you begin to tackle the challenge of pesticide use in your child's school? According to Bob McClintock. it all begins with educating the educators. First, find out what your school is using and when. States vary on what information is posted or sent home with a child. Ask. "Start talking to the administration in the school," advises McClintock. "Every school will be a little different. See how much they know about Integrated Pest Management (IPM)."

As far as cost goes, McClintock says the cost of using Tvedten and his nontoxic methods has been about the same as what the district was paying for chemical applications. But beyond the matter of dollars and cents, there's also "the value of having clean air in your school. Are we providing a better atmosphere for our students and staff? Yes, we are."

To learn about the laws in your state regarding pesticide use in schools, you can also check a database of more than 400 school districts that have implemented policies that reduce, ban, or inform about pesticide use. (Under a recently enacted New Jersey law, for instance, school officials must notify every parent and staff member seventy-two hours in advance, and students are not permitted back on school grounds for seven hours after a pesticide is applied.) To do this, go to the National Coalition Against the Misuse of Pesticides (NCAMP) at www.beyondpesticides.org and choose the "Children and Schools" section from the "programs" drop-down box.

DEGREES OF DANGER

While all chemical pesticides are poisons, not all pesticides are created equal, and the question of just how we may be affected by the residues of these various substances remaining in our food is still a long way from being answered. Then there's the matter of what can happen when we're directly exposed to them. One of the most widely applied chemicals, methyl bromide, is considered so dangerous that it's allowed to be used only by licensed professionals, and even so, it has left a mounting list of casualties (both dead and injured) in its wake.

Serial Killer in a Canister

For the Schemmel children—Derek, nine; Garrett, six; and their younger sister, Heidi, three—seeing their house surrounded by this "big old tent" was "all kind of exciting," recalled their mother, Anne. So much so, in fact, that she even took snapshots of each youngster at a different corner of the tented two-story, four-bedroom home she and her husband, Ken, had just purchased in Savannah, Georgia, after having relocated there from Illinois.

Many months after that September day in 1987, the sight of a similarly tented house around the corner "just sent this horrible chill up my whole body," Anne said.

Tenting their new home hadn't been the Schemmels' idea. A real estate agent had arranged it as a necessary precondition of the closing, the result of wood borers (termites) having been discovered during an inspection by Town & Country Extermination. The purpose of the tent was to allow the house to be fumigated with a chemical called methyl bromide, a procedure that would require the family to stay elsewhere "for a day or so."

To Anne Schemmel, a tent fumigation was a totally new experience. She even took a picture of the guard sitting out front. And while the sign posted on the lawn had warned people not to enter because a dangerous chemical was being used, never did she imagine that after the family had been assured it was perfectly safe to return, it could make them all sick—or would result in the death of her youngest child.

The first sign that something was amiss was when the family

returned on the evening of the day after the fumigation had been performed and noticed a "sickening sweet smell that seemed to be everywhere." After first opening the windows and then turning on the air-conditioning, they called the exterminating company, one of whose owners showed up the following day along with the real estate agent. The owner "really didn't make much of it, but did go around opening all the windows and turning the fans on high in order to air out the house," according to Anne. He also "offered to pay for us to go to a hotel that night." When asked if there was a problem with staying in the house, he replied, "Oh no, it's perfectly safe, you can stay."

The reason Anne stayed was that by this time, she "didn't even have the energy to pack or get out of bed . . . it was like I was in a daze, and if I wasn't throwing up, I was sleeping." Heidi, too, had started throwing up, and Derek was sent home from school early with similar symptoms. By the next day, however, Anne had recovered sufficiently to return to her teaching job, leaving her husband to care for Heidi. It was the following morning when Heidi refused to eat or drink that her mother began to fear she would become dehydrated and took her to see a general practitioner. He recommended that Heidi be taken to the local hospital, Memorial Medical Center.

It was there that Anne learned from a nurse that her daughter might have pneumonia, but she was told little else. "I told them . . . the house had been tented, and I asked them, 'Could that have caused it?' " she recalled. But no one there claimed to know anything about methyl bromide. "They'd never heard of it."

Eventually, Heidi was hooked up to an oxygen tent. Then, after she began gasping for air, she was moved to the pediatric intensive care unit. There, she had an emergency tracheotomy (a tube was inserted into her trachea to assist her breathing), and she was given continuous cardiopulmonary resuscitation (CPR) and open heart massage—but all to no avail. Finally, her mother was told the tragic news: "She's gone—we're so sorry; we don't know why she should have died." Months afterward, Anne learned that the nurses at the hospital had been terribly upset by her daughter's death, which was "the most horrible thing that ever happened to them. No one thought she was that sick." One of the pediatricians even visited the family and told them that "he had never seen anything like this in his life" and he needed to get some answers as to why it happened.

It took a local attorney, Jeff Lasky, however, to provide those answers a year after the little girl's death. Convinced that the fumigation was somehow responsible, he began his own investigation, finding out everything he could about methyl bromide—even attending classes and conventions for exterminators while posing as one—then trying to match up Heidi's symptoms with those he had read about. The result was a three-week civil trial—the longest in the county's history—in which an explanation finally emerged through the testimony of expert witnesses. First, it was established that the family had been told to return home far too soon, at least forty-eight hours being required for proper aeration of the house. It was also revealed how methyl bromide, an odorless gas, could react with other materials to produce new malodorous and toxic gases. Finally, it was established why Heidi alone had died: Methyl bromide gas had "pocketed" inside her plastic-covered mattress and in the drawers underneath, which the fumigators had failed to remove in advance. So convincing was the evidence that the jury wasted no time in reaching a verdict of wrongful death.

Despite winning her lawsuit, Anne remained deeply disturbed by the lack of public awareness of this toxic chemical that had claimed her daughter's life, at "how easily this can happen, how vulnerable everybody is." Seeking to share her experience with a wider audience, she contacted all the leading network talk shows, but got no response other than a "ready-made postcard" from Oprah Winfrey's show.

Today, there is far more awareness of methyl bromide, also known as bromomethane, than there was in the late 1980s. It has, in fact, been the subject of considerable controversy and an attempted phase-out since coming into the spotlight as a destroyer of the earth's protective ozone layer (at which it is regarded as fifty times more powerful than chlorine). Over the years, this most pernicious of poisons has also continued to be a virtual serial killer in a canister, striking down unsuspecting victims of all ages and in all walks of life, often gaining clandestine entry to their homes like a stealthy intruder in the night (and continuing to have no effective antidote, even when its effects are recognized). In less concentrated amounts, it has sickened hundreds of others, especially those living in the vicinity of agricultural fields where it has been used to fumigate the soil.

One might think all that would have been enough to warrant some type of decisive action to put this highly lethal pesticide out of commission. But that's been far from the case. In fact, the deferential treatment given by our government to this indiscriminate killer and ozone depleter reads like a case study of the influence of big contributors—in this case, big agribusiness interests—on the political process.

The sad fact is that had things gone as originally intended, methyl bromide would have been all but history by now, at least in the United States, where its production and importation were scheduled to end by the year 2001 under the Clean Air Act Amendments of 1990. Similarly, methyl bromide use should have been phased out on a global basis as well, under the Montreal Protocol of the United Nations Environment Programme.

But representatives of the agricultural sector cried foul, claiming that no viable substitute existed that was capable of killing so many pests—virtually everything with which it came in contact, in fact—and that banning it would put American food producers at an extreme disadvantage. And drumming up support for their position were not only various members of Congress to whose campaigns these interests had contributed, but none other than the USDA, whose own rules dictated that methyl bromide be used to fumigate a whole array of imported commodities. In fact, the late Edward Madigan, onetime secretary of agriculture, described it as "a very important chemical needed to sustain production and trade in agricultural commodities worldwide," the loss of which "would virtually stop international movement" of many such items.

With influential friends like that, methyl bromide's projected phase-out has been extended under the Clean Air Act to not take full effect until 2005, to coincide with an international phase-out for industrialized countries. (In developing nations, it won't be phased out until 2015.) But that may not really mean a great deal because not only are preshipment and quarantine uses exempt, but "critical and emergency uses" are allowed after that year, just as they are under amendments to the Montreal Protocol, which allows the chemical to keep being manufactured if there is "significant market disruption" without it.

Although there is no single replacement for methyl bromide, the United Nations Environment Programme's 1994 Report of the Methyl Bromide Technical Options Committee stated that for more than 90 percent of its current uses, there are alternatives, ones that either already exist or are in an advanced stage of development.

Methyl bromide, it should be noted, is not merely another toxic "spray." Rather, it is an invisible, odorless gas that can sequester itself in unexpected places, even seeping through pipes and air-conditioning ducts into adjoining spaces. Those sorts of things can happen during structural fumigations, which represent only a fraction of its use. Mostly, methyl bromide is used to sterilize the soil used to grow tomatoes, strawberries, and other crops. And while it is never used directly on crops under cultivation, it is often applied to harvested commodities, as well as in processed food plants, the idea being that any residues would soon disappear. But the discovery of methyl bromide residues in certain commodities, such as California nuts and Florida citrus, in the 1980s cast considerable doubt on that long-held supposition.

But why should all this concern you as a parent? Mainly because methyl bromide is still extensively used for a variety of purposes, and when it comes to toxic substances, it ranks right up there near the top of the list, in a category all by itself. Whereas other pesticides are still sources of concern (to which you and your kids should avoid being exposed whenever possible), exposure to methyl bromide can have far more dire and immediate consequences. At low levels, it can produce symptoms such as nausea, vomiting, vertigo, loss of muscle control, headaches, shortness of breath, and blurred vision. Beyond that, it can cause tremors, convulsions, delirium, respiratory failure, and central nervous system depression resulting in death. And—oh, yes—long-term exposure to small amounts may well be carcinogenic.

All of which means that, depending on where you live, your family may or may not be at risk of direct exposure to this deadly chemical. If you reside in the so-called Sunbelt, particularly in a place like Florida or California, your chances of encountering it are greatest. In that case, you need to be aware of tented structures and tarped fields (a tarp being an indicator that the soil is being fumigated). Treated areas are also not safe right after tents and tarps have been removed, since the gas is then vented into the surrounding environment.

Beyond that, do not let an exterminator talk you into using fumigation to get rid of an infestation (usually of termites). Instead, seek out nontoxic alternatives, such as heat and cold treatments. You might also talk to your neighbors about the dangers, and take precautions if one of them should have a fumigation in progress.

Then, too, if you're buying or renting a house in an agricultural area, it might be a good idea to avoid one that's close to farmland, as methyl bromide off-gassing from cultivated fields has at times sickened scores of neighbors. You might also want to examine the location of your children's school to determine its proximity to a farming area, and if there's one within a mile or two, perhaps you'll want to consider sending them to another facility.

You may also wish to inform your congressman of your concern about the hazards of continued methyl bromide use. But of course, the best way to discourage such a poison from being disseminated, and to avoid possible residues of it, is to buy organic food as often as possible.

One other thing: Because methyl bromide is a restricted-use substance, you're not likely to see your next-door neighbor out wielding a canister of it (that is, unless your neighbor happens to be licensed to use it). But the fact that it's for "professional use only" is no guarantee that it won't be used in a careless or negligent manner, as Anne Schemmel learned to her profound regret. To her, it's "unbelievable" that the company that applied it to her home should know so little about its hazards, or that "someone so irresponsible" should be "handling something so dangerous."

Toxic Tolerances

> Safe. *Adjective.* Not dangerous; unlikely to cause or result in harm, injury, or damage.

If you're like most of us, you probably assume that when the EPA allows a pesticide to be registered and used (for food, lawn care, or control of termites, for instance), it has officially declared that pesticide to be "safe." But at the EPA, the word "safe" isn't even in the vocabulary. According to Antonio Bravo, of the EPA's Office of Pesticide and Toxicology, "There is no definition for safe. There is a definition for what would be considered adverse (i.e., having an adverse effect on people) but not safe." The EPA, according to Bravo, "intentionally avoids [that] definition."

"No pesticide is 100 percent safe," adds Bravo. "Anybody in this agency would back me on that because pesticides . . . are designed to kill something, so how could they be safe? It runs counter to intuition."[12]

But while the agency won't say "safe," it does set tolerances—the legal limits of pesticides allowed as residues in food. "What a tolerance is supposed to indicate is a 'no effect level,'" comments Daniel Swartz, executive director of the Children's Environmental Health Network. "The only way that we could possibly have data that would give us absolute certainty of safety is to run scientific experiments in thousands of kids; the second way is that we don't use any of these things at all. I certainly don't opt for the first."[13]

To set a tolerance (which is in reality an "enforcement tool"), the EPA reviews animal studies designed to look for different types of organ damage (such as brain, reproductive, and liver damage) to the test animal, then divides the no-observable-effect level by an "uncertainty factor" of 100. But no matter how sophisticated the studies, they still deal with animals. "In the science of toxicology, recognizing anything we recommend with respect to these levels is based on extrapolation from models and animal studies," says Bravo. "There's a lot of gray area there."

To comply with the Food Quality Protection Act (see Chapter 1), regulators divide the established tolerance for a particular pesticide on a commodity—say, a tomato—by an additional safety factor of ten (unless they believe a lesser safety factor will do). Given the distinct lack so far of new neurotoxicity data that the law was designed to elicit, one might assume that such a factor would automatically go into effect for the majority of pesticides that have been reviewed. But that, as it turns out, is far from the case.

True, there have been some chemicals for which the added tenfold safety margin (or an even greater one) has been ordered, among them 12 of 39 of the organophosphates looked at. But by September 2000, only a quarter of the 105 chemicals reviewed had been assigned such safety factors, with the tolerances of another 22 percent multiplied by three. The remaining 53 percent, including 15 organophosphates, were allowed to retain their existing tolerances.

"The EPA has gotten them off the hook about 75 percent of the time without industry having to do a thing," is the way Richard Wiles, senior vice president of the Washington, DC–based Environmental Working Group, sums up the situation.[14]

But perhaps that's a reflection of the kind of pressure constantly affecting EPA personnel involved in the reappraisal. "On any individual pesticide," says Swartz, "the audience that is going to be most concerned and pay most attention is always going to be industry. They have the most at stake for any individual decision. The public may be worried about pesticides in general, but we're not going to spend hours going through the report on a particular pesticide. On the individual decisions that end up having the cumulative effect of setting the regulatory system, EPA faces certainly a lot more scrutiny and pressure from the folks who want to sell this stuff than from those who might be concerned [about its safety]."

Despite that, there has been progress made under the FPQA in providing better regulation of some of the most toxic pesticides, Wiles acknowledges, and perhaps even more than in other EPA programs. It's just that the pace of reform under the law is a far cry from any assumption consumers might make that the law ensures "safe" tolerances for pesticides in food.

"Safe is too abstract a term," is how Bravo puts it. "What we might call safe today may prove to be unsafe tomorrow . . . Too often people ask us—especially food processors—to declare that, say, avocados treated with this and that are safe. How could they be safe? You're using a killing agent on them. We could assess whether consumption of that avocado might result in some type of harmful effect to the consumer, but we could never say it's safe."

The Hidden Hazard of Flying Your Family "Down Under"

It was only an hour or two into a flight home to Los Angeles from Sydney, Australia, that the wife and thirteen-year-old grandson of Dr. Richard Dorazio, chief of surgery of the Southern California Kaiser Permanente Medical Group, began to feel ill. At the same time, Dr. Dorazio became aware of "a strong smell of pesticide," which lasted throughout the flight.

The source of that smell became clear to Dr. Dorazio shortly after a flight attendant inquired about his wife's condition. From her, he learned that the plane had been sprayed and that crew members had been experiencing similar problems. He later expressed concern in a complaint to the airline that her symptoms and those of his grandson were "the result of chemical toxicity."

The spraying, however, wasn't the airline's idea. Such pesticide application, called "disinsection," is the result of a government policy in Australia and several other countries intended to make sure no alien bugs arrive via aircraft. Some years ago, in fact, spraying aircraft cabins with pesticides, including DDT, with passengers aboard was common practice in the United States. But it was dropped after the CDC found it to be neither safe nor effective.

It took considerable publicity and pressure from the U.S. Department of Transportation to get most of the two or three dozen countries that required disinsection (with a chemical labeled as "hazardous to humans" and not to be inhaled or to come in contact with eyes or skin) before passengers could disembark to also drop the policy. But a few, including Australia and New Zealand, have continued to require it. (For a list of the countries that require spraying, see page 129.)

As an alternative to exposing passengers directly, airlines flying in and out of those countries have switched to a method called "residual spraying," which calls for permeating a plane's interior surfaces with a long-lasting insecticide at eight-week intervals while neither passengers nor crew members are on board. The spray, applied by workers in protective gear, is permethrin, a possible carcinogen that the EPA doesn't allow to be used in aircraft cabins in the United States.

Perhaps it should come as no surprise, then, that chronic adverse reactions have been suffered by flight attendants, some of whom have resorted to legal action. And as Dr. Dorazio and others have discovered, passengers may also be affected during long flights, a factor that should be taken into consideration before putting one's family (particularly small children) on an airliner to one of these destinations (especially if anyone in your family is asthmatic or sensitive to chemicals, in which case it might be preferable to take a "slow boat").

STRATEGIES FOR LIMITING YOUR EXPOSURE

Toxic pesticides may seem impossible to avoid, but that doesn't mean you can't cut down substantially on the amounts to which you and your family are exposed. It's simply a matter of knowing where you're most apt to encounter them and having a resistance plan in place. Following are a number of things you can do to reduce exposure and keep your kids as safe as possible:

- Buy certified organic food whenever you can.
- Recognize that reducing pesticide risk begins at home by finding alternative methods of pest control. (Bringing in professional exterminators, for instance, does not guarantee that pesticide use in your home will be any safer. In fact, it might actually have the opposite effect, as commercial applicators often use more potent chemicals than are available to homeowners, such as methyl bromide.)
- If you live in an apartment, don't automatically accept a policy of having to give maintenance personnel entry to apply pesticides. Read Chapter 5 for alternative methods and request that one or more of these be implemented. If the apartment owner still insists on spraying, you may wish to seek assistance in invoking your right not to have your family exposed to toxic chemicals. If spraying does occur, try to leave your house for a day or so, and keep the kids away for as long as possible. Think about sending them to a friend or relative's house for the weekend if the spraying is done on a Friday. Remember, even if you rent, your home is still your castle!
- Don't allow flea collars on any dogs or cats in your house, as the chemicals will also deposit themselves on your carpet,

sofa, bed, and any other place that the animal inhabits. Also, keep in mind that children tend to hug and kiss pets, which results in direct exposure. (In other words, if you wouldn't put a flea collar on your child, don't put one on your pet.)

- Instruct your children about the dangers of playing on grass that has been sprayed, and caution them to look for the flags planted by applicators. You may also want to be on the lookout for brown and withered weeds, another indicator of pesticide use.

- Avoid using shampoos or treatments for head lice on your child, as they may contain a toxic organophosphate insecticide. (See Chapter 5 for alternative treatment options.)

- Find out if and when your kids' school or day-care facility will be treated with pesticides. Discuss the dangers of exposing kids to toxic chemicals with teachers and administrators, and the possibilities of using alternative techniques such as Integrated Pest Management (IPM), a system that combines such methods as biological controls, pest monitoring, and habitat manipulation with prudent use of the least toxic pesticides available. Some professional pest control companies specialize in IPM. (Don't just count on school officials notifying you about pesticide applications; make sure you ask them to.)

- If you use well water, have it tested for pesticide contamination as well as toxic metals such as lead.

- To avoid tracking pesticides onto your carpet, where they can be picked up by toddlers or small children, take off your shoes upon entering the house.

- Flying to certain international destinations will expose you to many hours in a pesticide-treated cabin. The governments of Australia and New Zealand, to name two, require that planes be treated with either an aerosol pesticide while passengers are present or a stronger, long-lasting residual spray in empty cabins. Neither are allowed by law to be used in the United States (which is why planes are treated elsewhere), and the residual has caused serious health problems

FLYING IN THE FOG

A number of countries continue to require the use of either an aerosol or residual pesticide in the passenger cabin of airplanes. While the list has grown considerably shorter over the past five years, it's doubtful that the remaining countries, especially Australia, will change their policy. Even airlines that use the residual method (spraying while the aircraft is empty) can *still* use an aerosol pesticide spray while passengers are on board if the plane's certification period (the time during which the pesticide is considered effective) has expired or if requested by local authorities.

As of this writing, the following countries require residual pesticide application while passengers are not on board:

Australia	Jamaica
Barbados	New Zealand
Fiji	

Panama requires aerosol pesticide application while passengers are not on board.

The following countries require aerosol pesticide application while passengers *are* on board:

Grenada	Madagascar
India	Trinidad and Tobago
Kiribati	Uruguay

The following countries require pesticide application (most likely aerosol) on certain flights while passengers are on board:

Czech Republic—flights from areas where contagious diseases are present

Indonesia—flights from areas where infectious diseases are present

South Africa—flights from areas where malaria or yellow fever are present

Switzerland—flights from Intertropical Africa

United Kingdom—flights from countries where malaria is present in flight attendants repeatedly exposed to it. Since you can't avoid exposure once on board, you may want to reconsider a trip to these destinations, especially if you are asthmatic, chemically sensitive, or traveling with a child or infant.

With so many pesticides being casually sold over the counter and applied in locales ranging from urban apartments to suburban lawns to farm fields, it's easy to be lulled into accepting the chemical lobbies' claims that they're really designed only to kill insects, weeds, and rodents, and not to be injurious to people. But one need look no further than the disaster that took place in Bhopal, India, in 1984, when a cloud of toxic gas from a Union Carbide plant that manufactured pesticide ingredients killed thousands of people and incapacitated numerous others, to realize how perilously foolish such acceptance is.

There's no getting around the facts that these chemicals are intended to destroy living organisms, and that even "tiny" amounts bioaccumulate in our bodies, reacting with other toxic residues in ways still not completely understood. Perhaps most important, it's well established that kids are apt to be adversely affected by these poisons far more than adults. That's why we must do everything within our power to keep these poisons not only out of the "reach" of children, but out of their diets and environments as well.

RESOURCES

Pesticides and Other Environmental Toxins

Environmental Research Foundation (ERF)
Web site: www.rachel.org
    Scientific data on the effects toxic substances have on human health and the environment.

Environmental Working Group (EWG)
Web site: www.ewg.org
    Information, articles, and reports related to pesticides, drinking water, air pollution, food contamination, and environmental laws.

National Pesticide Information Center (NPIC)
Telephone: 800-858-7378
Web site: http://npic.orst.edu
    Facts on the health effects of pesticides, their environmental impact, and related federal regulations.

U.S. Public Interest Research Group (PIRG) Online
Web site: www.uspirg.org
    The Web site of U.S. PIRG, a public-interest watchdog organization that specializes in investigative research, media exposés, advocacy, and litigation to protect public interests against special interests.

Pesticides in Aircraft (Disinsection)

Department of Transportation
Web site: http://ostpxweb.dot.gov/policy/safety/disin.htm
    Information about aircraft pesticide spraying, as well as contact names and numbers for airlines.

Journalists Linda and Bill Bonvie
Web site: www.kefir.net/spray/
    Articles by Linda and Bill Bonvie on aircraft pesticide spraying, as well as a short video showing how the residual pesticide is applied.

Making Your Home a Nontoxic Haven

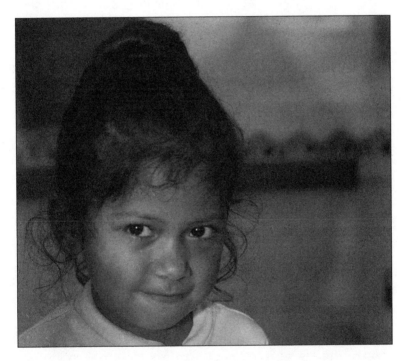

"Children today face hazards that were neither known nor imagined a few decades ago."
— Philip J. Landrigan et al., "Children's Health and the "Environment: A New Agenda for Prevention Research," *Environmental Health Perspectives*, volume 106, supplement 3, June 1998

WHAT YOU'LL FIND IN THIS CHAPTER

Commonly used cleaning agents pose significant risks to kids. Accidental poisonings aren't the only way cleaning agents can harm children. Keeping them locked up isn't enough; when you use them, even according to the label instructions, you're creating a potential toxic exposure. The long-term effects are not required to be listed on the label. And the fact that something is sold in a store does not make it automatically safe. Commonly used products can cause nerve damage, reproductive damage, cancer, and respiratory problems. Check out our list of nontoxic alternatives for better ways to clean.

Is your lawn a safe place on which to play? Pesticides and herbicides don't belong where children play. Frequently used herbicides such as products containing the chemical 2,4-D (which was a component of Agent Orange) have been found to significantly increase the risk of certain cancers in people and dogs. Why not make your lawn a safe haven for kids instead of a toxic waste dump? See our recommendations for safe grass on your home turf.

Risk-free indoor pest control is not only possible, but a lot easier than you might think. Find out how to keep your home free of insects and vermin without resorting to toxic sprays and deadly fumigants with some help from an expert in the field.

A real reason to be afraid of the dark and the damp is toxic mold. It's a microscopic monster that can invade your home wherever there's a leak, and it thrives in damp and dark places. True, it may not have been concocted in a laboratory, but it can make your family quite ill nevertheless—and has been known to drive people out of their homes.

Chemical sensitivity, can be an end result of toxic overload. When your body has had all it can stand of exposure to noxious substances, the result could well be an intolerance to all chemicals, even to everyday ones like detergent and fragrances. This is another good reason to keep your kids as chemical-free as possible in today's world.

The late humorist Erma Bombeck once offered the following advice about housework: "If the item doesn't multiply, smell, catch on fire or block the refrigerator door, let it be." But if you cook and have children, pets, or both, messes and smells that you can't simply ignore are an inevitable part of everyday life. You've simply got to clean. The question is, how can you best manage those messes without jeopardizing your family's health or safety?

TOXIC CLEANING AGENTS: UNHEALTHIER THAN DIRT

As we're looking for shortcuts to better enable us to clean, scrub, and remove stains, we're also stocking our cupboards with an alarming array of toxic substances that, among other things, can cause respiratory problems and damage the nervous system, kidneys, skin, and eyes. While commercials may show happy kids dancing down the street in super-white clothes and bouquets of flowers blossoming from plug-in air fresheners, what they don't discuss are the hazards inherent in these chemical cleaning agents.

The most obvious risk from household cleaning products, of course, is that of accidental poisoning. But simply keeping cleaners out of a child's reach doesn't necessarily mean the child is shielded from dangerous toxic exposures. Don't expect labeling to tell the whole story, either. Key words such as "caution" refer only to immediate hazards. Potential long-term effects are not required to be listed on the packaging.[1] A study by the U.S. Consumer Product Safety Commission on home chemicals found more than 150 that are linked to allergies, birth defects, cancer, or psychological abnormalities.

Fortunately, there are effective alternatives available, and they're a lot easier to substitute for commercial chemical cleaners than you might think. After all, before consumers were lured by the promise of scrubbing bubbles, dancing detergents, and pine-scented floor cleaners, they somehow did manage to keep things clean and fresh-smelling. Your home and clothes can likewise be scrubbed and deodorized using today's labor-saving appliances, but without having to resort to toxic and often caustic cleaning liquids and powders. For a list of some of these safer alternatives, see Table 5.1.

TABLE 5.1
Safer Alternatives to Toxic Cleaning Agents

Instead of . . .	Why not try . . .
Chlorine bleach. The most common accidentally swallowed cleaning agent is bleach. Chlorine is a lung and eye irritant. In addition, when chlorine is mixed with ammonia or another acidic cleaning agent, even vinegar, a highly toxic gas is released.	Nonchlorine dry bleach or a hydrogen peroxide–based liquid bleach.
Dishwashing detergent. Phosphates that end up in lakes, rivers, estuaries, and oceans after they go down your drain act as fertilizers, causing algae to grow faster, which then pollutes the water.	A vegetable oil–based soap for hand-washing dishes or an automatic dishwasher soap that's low in phosphates, such as Seventh Generation brand.
Drain cleaner. Drain cleaners are among the most dangerous products you can bring into your home. They are corrosive and can cause blindness if splashed in the eyes and chemical burns if swallowed.	The easiest method of preventing a clogged drain: a strainer. Most bathroom sinks get clogged by hair.
	Cleaning the drain with a long, thin plastic device with sharp "hair catchers" running up the sides, available in hardware stores. Work it down into the drain and slowly pull it out. It may take several tries, but it does work well. (Keep it away from kids, however, as it's sharp.)

Instead of . . .	Why not try . . .
	Pouring a handful of baking soda and ½ cup of vinegar down the drain, then covering the drain for 15 minutes to seal in the carbon dioxide gas. The bubbles should loosen the clog. Rinse with 2 quarts of boiling water and follow with a plunger.
Furniture polish. Many furniture polishes contain petroleum distillates, which are very dangerous if swallowed.	Polishing unvarnished wood surfaces with almond, walnut, or olive oil. Work the oil in well, then wipe off the excess, as oily surfaces attract dirt.
	Polishing varnished wood with a mild vegetable oil soap.
	Revitalizing old furniture with linseed oil.
	Washing painted wood with a mixture of 1 teaspoon of washing soda and 1 gallon of hot water. Rinse with clear water.
	Removing watermarks from wood furniture by rubbing toothpaste on the spot and polishing with a soft cloth.
Oven cleaner. Conventional oven cleaners are among the most dangerous of household products, since they are corrosive and can cause chemical burns if accidentally swallowed.	Mixing 1 part vinegar with about 4 parts water in a spray bottle. Spray onto the cool oven surface and scrub. Use baking soda or a citrus-based cleaner on stubborn spots.

Instead of . . .	Why not try . . .
	Mixing together in a spray bottle 2 tablespoons of liquid soap (not detergent), 2 teaspoons of borax, and enough warm water to fill the bottle. Make sure the borax completely dissolves to avoid clogging the squirter. Spray on the mixture, holding the bottle very close to the oven surface; leave on for 20 minutes; then scrub with steel wool and a nonchlorine scouring powder.
	A nonchlorinated powder such as Bon Ami or a combination of baking soda and salt mixed into a paste with water.
Toilet bowl cleaner. Avoid solid toilet bowl deodorizers that contain paradichlorobenzene, a chemical that causes cancer in animals. Also watch out for acid-containing toilet bowl cleaners, which should never be mixed with anything containing chlorine.	Pouring in 1 cup of borax mixed with ½ cup of white vinegar and leaving it overnight (be sure to close the lid to keep out thirsty pets and curious kids).
	Removing stains with a paste of lemon juice and borax. Let the paste sit for about 20 minutes, then scrub the stain with a bowl brush.
Tub and sink cleaner.	A nonchlorinated cleanser such as Bon Ami.

Instead of . . .	Why not try . . .
	Removing tough stains with a citrus-based cleaner used at full strength (not diluted.)
	Baking soda, which is abrasive.
	Removing mineral deposits around faucets by covering them with strips of paper towels soaked in vinegar. Let the strips sit for 1 hour and then wash the porcelain.

Source: Enviroene, a part of the Environmental Protection Agency Web site (http://es.epa.gov).

Just What Do You Mean by "Clean" Anyway?

What does "clean" smell like to you? Does it smell like pine or lemon or even ammonia? Stop and think about it for a moment. "Clean" is actually the absence of something undesirable, be it scum, mold, germs, or cookie crumbs on the couch. Something that smells "clean," then, should actually have no smell at all. But led on by advertisers, we tend to associate the concept of "clean" with various synthetic masking fragrances, smells that are actually a form of air pollution in disguise.

"We've been programmed to believe it's only clean if it smells clean," says Elizabeth Sword, executive director of the Children's Health Environmental Coalition (CHEC). As a result, she says, "clean" for most people has come to mean "lemon or piney fresh; it has to have an odor. Nobody stops to think that the odor is a chemical."

You may think that by locking up such cleaning products, you're protecting your children. But what happens when you take them from behind the locked cabinet and use them the way they're designed to be used? "When you apply these chemicals to the floor surface, the high chair tray, the crib, anywhere else that your child is coming into contact with the surface, the child is still exposed," Sword points out.

If you spray your countertops with a chemical agent, it may eliminate most microorganisms, but the chances are pretty high that it will also coat those surfaces with an invisible toxic residue. But isn't that what it takes to protect against germs and dangerous pathogens such as salmonella and *E. coli?* No, it might actually require far simpler protective methods. Instead of "nuking" all your kitchen surfaces with toxic chemicals, for instance, why not simply use a special board for raw meat and one for veggies that can go in the dishwasher?

It seems that in our quest to sanitize our environment, we've grouped all "germs" together and don't bother to discriminate between those that can really do us harm and those that can't. Like insects, some microorganisms are genuinely beneficial and help us fight harmful germs, or pathogens, but strong chemical cleaners simply zap both kinds.

In fact, recent evidence suggests that exposure to a certain amount of germs at an early age might actually make children less subject to allergies and asthma. A study published in September 2002 in the *New England Journal of Medicine* found that European farm children exposed to twice as many endotoxins—that is, bits of bacterial cell walls from farm animals and other sources—as nonfarm kids had far lower rates of common, or atopic, asthma and hay fever. In either case, those exposed to more germs from bedding dust had about half the risk of asthma and 60 percent as much for hay fever. That study, which jibed with the results of another involving pet exposure in the first year of life (discussed later in this chapter), tends to bear out a recent theory called the hygienic hypothesis, which holds that early contact with some germs tends to bolster the immune system against allergies.

Treating children's toys and household items such as cutting boards with a pesticide to reduce the growth of bacteria and other germs is unnecessary at best. At worst, it could trigger allergic reactions, kill beneficial bacteria, contribute to an increase in antibiotic-resistant microorganisms, and reduce whatever level of immunity that exposure to germs might help children develop. The active ingredient in Microban, a pesticide incorporated into numerous items, such as cutting boards, humidifiers, and even socks, is triclosan, which the FDA has been studying for more than twenty-five years. Several years ago, companies started claiming that toys containing the chemical helped safeguard toddlers against infectious diseases. A subsequent agreement between the manufacturers and the EPA stipulated that playthings treated with Microban can no longer be advertised as protecting kids' health. Such a claim, the agency feared, could mislead parents into abandoning basic hygienic precautions, the best one still being hand-washing.

Unfortunately, such fundamental old-fashioned hygiene also hasn't been spared the toxic influence of the chemical industry. It seems almost impossible these days to find hand soap that does not contain an antibacterial agent. But isn't that good for kids? After all, they are always putting their hands in their mouth, so why not kill the germs?

True, it may be killing germs all right, but not always the right ones. In the process, it may be doing away with beneficial bacteria that actually help protect us against harmful pathogens. Then, too, like the triclosan-treated products, routine use of antibacterial soaps could create stronger, tougher versions of disease-causing microbes and actually help them to flourish. The same is true when you clean surfaces with antibacterial cleaners. So save the heavy ammunition for times when it may really be needed. Remember: When it comes to basic cleaning, unadulterated soap and water is still the best idea.

"It's not a question of cleaning any differently, it's a question of cleaning with something different," says Sword. "You can still wash your floors, but reconsider what you wash them with." By using chemical-based cleaning products, she maintains, while you may not see an immediate adverse effect on your child, "you may set the stage for a negative outcome later on."

THE TOXIC TRIO: SAY ADIOS TO THESE, PRONTO!

Corrosive cleaning products pose serious dangers of ingestion, inhalation, and skin burns to both children and pets. Swallowing even a small amount of such a caustic substance can seriously injure the mouth, stomach, and esophagus. Don't allow your home to be a place that harbors this trio of toxic hazards:

- Drain cleaners
- Oven cleaners
- Acid-based toilet bowl cleaners

How Much Are You Contributing to Your Own Indoor Air-Pollution Index?

Then there's the often overlooked issue of the air quality inside your home, your own indoor "air-pollution index," so to speak. Like office buildings that are constructed to be more energy efficient, our homes tend to retain indoor pollutants in their ambient air, especially in winter, when windows are kept shut. Since most people spend about 90 percent of their time indoors, kids and adults with asthma and chemical sensitivities may be especially affected. EPA studies have found indoor air-pollution levels may be two to five times higher, and occasionally more than a hundred times higher, than outdoor levels.[2]

Indoor Air: A Gathering Place for Irritants

A lot of families wouldn't dream of living near a chemical plant belching toxic fumes, yet continually pollute the air inside their homes with a variety of noxious chemicals emitted by the products they use for cleaning surfaces, clothes, appliances, and carpets; painting the walls; waxing the floors; and "freshening" the air. Volatile organic compounds (VOCs), many of which are known to cause cancer in animals and humans, can be released simply by using, and to a lesser extent storing, common household products. For example:

- Extremely hazardous VOCs such as toluene, styrene, xylene, and trichloroethylene can be "off-gassed" from a variety of sources, such as dry-cleaned clothing, spot removers, floor waxes and polishes, air fresheners, glues, paints, varnishes, and art supplies. Trichloroethylene was one of the chemicals suspected of causing a cluster of childhood leukemia cases from contaminated drinking water in Woburn, Massachusetts. The lawsuit against the companies that polluted the town was the subject of the 1998 movie *A Civil Action*.
- Xylene, ketones, and aldehydes are VOCs contained in many aerosols and air fresheners. In one study, babies under six months who lived in homes where air fresheners were used frequently had 30 percent more ear infections than babies who were exposed less frequently. Xylene may cause birth defects.
- EPA studies have shown that while using products containing VOCs, you expose yourself and others to very high levels of pollution, and these high concentrations remain in the air a long time after use.

One of the first things to remember is that just because a product is sold in your favorite store, it is not automatically safe to use, especially around children. A child's ability to excrete toxic substances has not fully developed. Exposures that have little impact on an adult can significantly harm a child. The younger a child is, the greater the potential for permanent or long-lasting damage. Children simply do not have the same capacity to detoxify as adults and are therefore more susceptible to the adverse effects of indoor chemicals.

While there are a variety of factors that might contribute to your indoor air-pollution index, the biggest could well be a misguided attempt on your part to create a "clean" and "fresh" environment with unnecessary chemical agents.

Tips for Improving Indoor Air Quality

- Ventilate your home more frequently. Something as simple as opening the window can help significantly in removing pollutants from your home environment. (If your neighbors use pesticides outside, try to find out when and keep windows shut during those times.) Proper ventilation is especially important if you have recently painted, installed new carpeting, or renovated.
- Avoid the use of aerosol sprays. If they are absolutely necessary, don't store them—or for that matter, any other cleaning agents and detergents—under the kitchen sink, as many people do. It's best to keep them in the garage or laundry room, or in some other area where they won't be within such easy reach of your kids.
- Avoid using air fresheners, both aerosols and plug-in types.
- Don't use pesticides indoors (or outdoors, for that matter).
- Avoid dry-cleaning your clothing. Dry-cleaned items release highly toxic chemicals, especially when they are in an enclosed environment such as your car or closet. If you do dry-clean your clothes, remove the plastic cover as soon as possible (making sure to discard it) and hang the item outside for an hour or two. This will help to vent the fumes from any dry-cleaning chemicals such as trichloroethylene, so that toxic levels of these gases won't build up in your home.
- Get the biggest welcome mat you can find. A doormat will help keep particles picked up on shoes, such as dust and pesticides, from getting inside. In addition, we recommend removing your shoes upon entering your home, so as not to track in these substances from outside.
- When painting, look for low-odor, latex, water-based paints. Paint only on days when you can open all the windows and fully ventilate the house. If possible, keep your children out of the house during painting and for a day or two afterward, perhaps making arrangements for them to stay with a friend or relative.

VINYL: THE PLASTIC WITH A BAD RECORD

Polyvinyl chloride (PVC), also known as vinyl and once used to make phonograph records, is bad from start to finish. Because it uses chlorine, the PVC manufacturing process produces dioxin, still considered the most toxic synthetic substance there is. PVC also produces dioxin when it's burned.

Since PVC is hard and brittle, making it into toys and other products involves adding various toxic ingredients and stabilizers, including lead and cadmium, as well as substantial amounts of chemical softeners known as phthalates. Both industry-sponsored and government testing found that the softeners may cause serious health effects ranging from liver and kidney damage to reproductive problems. Subsequent studies conducted in 1997 by Greenpeace found that the chemicals in PVC could easily leak into children's mouths.

Due to pressure from both consumers and consumer advocacy groups (with most of the pressure coming from Greenpeace), the U.S. Consumer Product Safety Commission (CPSC) requested that toy manufacturers stop using lead, phthalates, and cadmium in vinyl toys and other objects meant to be put in a child's mouth, such as pacifiers and teething rings. Since the CPSC action is just a "request," however, making mouth toys without PVC plastic is strictly voluntary. Some manufacturers have chosen to eliminate PVC entirely, others just in mouth toys, and others just in toys for children under three. Since kids tend to put almost anything in their mouth, it's best to banish PVC-made toys and other products entirely (especially PVC nipples and pacifiers). There are many alternatives, and with consumer pressure still on, it's likely more and more companies will banish PVC over the coming years.

For an update on products that are PVC-free, go to the Greenpeace 2000 report card for toy manufacturers and retailers at http://greenpeaceusa.org/features/reportcard2000text.htm.

- Use ventilating fans in the bathroom and kitchen. If you have a gas stove, try to get as much ventilation in the kitchen as possible. According to William J. Rea, M.D., of the Environmental Health Center in Dallas, Texas, one of the most significant sources of indoor air pollution is cooking with gas, due to the incomplete combustion products it generates.

- Consider getting one or more portable air purifiers. An air purifier with a HEPA filter can help reduce levels of animal dander, dust, pollen, and cooking odors. A machine of this sort will purify all the air in a room in a given period of time, depending on the room size.
- Reduce fireplace use. While cozy and warm, fireplaces greatly increase indoor air pollution. And since you usually use a fireplace during the winter, closed windows keep contamination levels high. Never burn printed paper or particleboard. Keep in mind that children who live in homes where the fireplace is frequently used are more susceptible to upper respiratory and ear infections.

YOUR NOSE KNOWS? NOT ALWAYS

Just because you can't smell it doesn't necessarily mean it's not there or not hazardous to your health and even potentially lethal. Carbon monoxide, for example, is odorless, yet can kill you within a relatively short time, which is why it's so important to have working carbon monoxide detectors and to keep your home well ventilated. Radon gas, which can seep into a house through a crack in the foundation, is also odorless, but can have deadly long-term consequences. In fact, it accounts for more than 20,000 lung cancer deaths a year, which is why radon testing is also recommended.

The same concept applies to many pesticides that are applied in the home. We might not always be able to smell them, but they can still have highly toxic effects on our bodies.

WHAT'S WARM AND FUZZY, AND MAY ACTUALLY HELP REDUCE ALLERGIES?

It's a concern with which we're all familiar, especially if you have a new infant in the house: Will the pet dog or cat trigger allergies and/or asthma in the baby? Should you find a new home for the pet you've had for years? You may have been told by doctors and concerned in-laws that a house with animals is a bad environment for a baby.

But what if the truth is often just the opposite?

It now appears that may well be the case. According to recent studies conducted in the United States and abroad, exposure during infancy to two or more pets in the house may actually decrease a child's susceptibility to allergies and asthma while growing up.

In the latest such study, chronicled in the *Journal of the American Medical Association*, researchers kept tabs on some 474 Detroit-area children from birth to the ages of six or seven. At that point, slightly more than a third of those whose families had no cats or dogs during their first year of life had developed skin sensitivity to six common irritants, including dust mites and pollen. For those exposed to a single cat or dog, the figure was slightly higher. However, it dropped to 15 percent among the 78 children whose homes had at least two pets.

Similar results were seen in testing for blood markers that indicated sensitivity to any of seven allergens. After the results were adjusted for factors that might contribute to allergic reactions, such as exposure to cigarette smoke or dust mites and a parental history of asthma, the risk of allergies dropped between 67 and 77 percent for a child whose household contained two or more pets.

Dr. Thomas Platts-Mills, an allergy expert at the University of Virginia who published an earlier study showing that exposure to cats can help protect against allergies, estimated that as many as 20 percent of people develop tolerance to pet allergens by living with animals, something he referred to as a "big phenomenon."

Some children who might otherwise be allergic, Dr. Platts-Mills noted, don't become allergic to a cat living in the house with them. "That's very important," he said, "because it implies that high-dose natural exposure can give rise to a form of tolerance."

Dr. Dennis Owenby, an allergist at the Medical College of Georgia who led the Detroit-area study, said his group theorized that children's immune systems may actually be bolstered by exposure to irritants that animals track in from outside. If so, it would jibe with the growing viewpoint that our focus on maintaining an overly clean, antiseptic environment is actually somewhat responsible for the current rise in allergies and asthma cases.

Dr. Magaziner, however, cautions that exposure to pets will probably not help children who have already been diagnosed with allergies to animals, and that such kids are probably better off continuing to avoid contact with animals. In such cases, classical allergy symptoms such as sneezing, nasal congestion, sinus headache, and itchy, watery eyes may be triggered by contact with a dog or cat, possibly at a friend's house, and steps should be taken to limit that exposure.

CREATING A POISON-FREE ZONE IN YOUR OWN BACKYARD

"Why don't you and your friends go out in the yard and play" is one of the most common requests that kids, especially those living in suburbia, are apt to hear from busy and distracted parents. But all too often these days, that innocent-sounding admonition may be compromising children's health in ways that usually conscientious moms and dads may never even have contemplated.

When Kids Become "Collateral Damage" in the War on Weeds

Is there a chemical arsenal stored in your garage, ready for an all-out assault on an invading enemy army? There very well may be, if you consider weeds and dandelions as alien forces requiring weapons of mass destruction to be eradicated from your turf. But before you decide that chemical warfare is called for in your pursuit of the Great American Lawn, you might want to take time out to consider whether such a cosmetic goal is worth putting the health and safety of your family in jeopardy. That green monotone you're so busy cultivating and defending is not, after all, really something representing the beauty of nature, but rather an unnatural veneer made possible by the chemical revolution (as well as an Englishman who invented the lawn mower in 1830).

As for your line of defense, keep in mind that just because a toxic chemical is used outside doesn't make it any safer. In fact, kids may have even more direct exposure to lawn chemicals than other kinds, given the way they're prone to roll and play in grass that, despite how green it looks, may have been recently contaminated with pesticides and herbicides. Do you really want your kids or their neighborhood friends to become "collateral damage" in the war you're waging against weeds?

One such poison, in fact, may not be all that far removed from a chemical agent used in actual combat. Agent Orange, which was applied extensively in Vietnam as a defoliant, was 50 percent 2,4-D, a common herbicide that is currently incorporated in many popular lawn-care products. More than 600 million pounds of 2,4-D are applied in the United States each year, by homeowners in their gardens and lawns, as well as by farmers to control weeds and to ensure that all their tomatoes ripen at the same time[3] and by railroad and highway departments to clear brush. The chemical has also been the subject of several health studies, one of which was done on dogs living in homes where products containing 2,4-D were used outside. The finding that those pets died of cancer at twice the expected rate[4] is remarkably similar to what was seen with farmers and railroad workers studied who applied the herbicide. The dogs had double the rate of malignant lymphomas and non-Hodgkin's lymphomas. (Non-Hodgkin's lymphoma has become the second fastest-growing cancer in people during the last fifteen years.) The farmers, who were studied in the Midwestern United States, Sweden, and Saskatchewan, Canada, had an increase of soft tissue sarcomas, malignant lymphomas, and non-Hodgkin's lymphomas.

Another popular weed killer, glyphosate (the active ingredient in Roundup), was identified in a 1993 report by the School of Public Health at the University of California, Berkeley, as the third most commonly reported cause of pesticide-related illness among farmworkers.

Considering the popularity of 2,4-D and glyphosate, suspect chemicals seem almost impossible to avoid. But one place you can manage to steer clear of them (as well as other pesticides and herbicides) is on your home turf, which is probably the place where your kids play the most anyway. Once again, keep in mind that a child, whose liver and excretion pathways have not yet matured, detoxifies far less efficiently than an adult. (Sweating, for instance, is one way that such poisons are eliminated and something children are less apt to do.) If you have pets that like to roll around in the grass, that's yet another reason to make your lawn a no-poison zone. Not only can chemical residues make your dog or cat sick, but they're likely to be brought into the house on your pet's paws and fur.

Ongoing exposure to lawn chemicals and pesticides can either cause acute reactions (when you know right away that something is wrong) or can develop into health problems years later, as seen in the studies on dogs and farmers.

One particularly drastic example of an acute reaction was seen in a patient of Dr. William Rea, a four-year-old girl who was eventually transferred to his Environmental Health Center in Dallas. After rolling and playing on a treated lawn for just a day, she started vomiting and developed a swelling in her left leg. At first admitted to a Florida hospital, she was thought to have a clot, but instead developed gangrene of her foot from her exposure to the lawn chemicals in which she played. Losing the tips of three toes, the girl also developed multiple sensitivities to food, pesticides, petrochemicals, and chlorine.

You can have a chemical-free lawn for your kids with probably less effort than it takes to properly apply these chemicals. For example, if you follow the label for a popular brand of 2,4-D–containing herbicide, whose package says that "controlling weeds in your lawn has never been easier," you'll be instructed to wear a long-sleeved shirt, long pants, socks, shoes, and rubber gloves—just right for yard work on a hot summer's day. You must rinse the gloves before removal, wash your hands with soap and water, and if any of the chemical has gotten onto your clothing, you must immediately remove and launder it separately.

If the way herbicides and pesticides are described in the EPA's flyer "Make a Call: Save a Life," below, makes you uneasy about what you're putting on your lawn, this might be a good time to go to the garage and trash your antiweed chemical arsenal. (Be sure to dispose of such chemicals properly; even though you're allowed to spray them over your lawn and garden, you're most likely not allowed to throw them in the trash because they are considered hazardous waste.)

Advising people to call the National Pesticide Telecommunications Network to learn how to "safely" use pesticides and herbicides, the EPA warns:

> Want to kill a bug . . . a weed . . . a rat? If you do it with a pesticide spray or powder, you are using a poison. Every time you use a poison, you need to know how to protect yourself and your family against misuse.
>
> Weed killers, bug sprays and rat baits work because they poison living things . . . There are thousands of pesticide poisonings each year. They cause severe rashes or nausea—sometimes permanent disability, occasionally death.

Ridding your home of poisons capable of causing everything from severe rashes and nausea to cancer, brain and nervous-system damage, and death is within your power. You don't have to ask for permission or convince anyone of their dangers; you're in charge here! Just saying "no" to home pesticide and herbicide use is one of the easiest ways to protect your kids from the risks inherent in these poisons.

The Fair-Haired Weed

"If dandelions were rare and fragile, people would knock themselves out to pay $14.95 a plant, raise them by hand in greenhouses, and form dandelion societies and all that. But, they are everywhere and don't need us and kind of do what they please. So we call them weeds and murder them at every opportunity," notes best-selling author Robert Fulghum in *All I Really Need to Know I Learned in Kindergarten* (G. K. Hall and Co., 1989).

The next time you see golden dandelions mingling with your grass, consider this:

- Dandelion greens contain vitamins A, C, and D, as well as iron, magnesium, lecithin, zinc, potassium, manganese, copper, and calcium.
- According to noted herbalist James A. Duke, Ph.D., dandelion roots and greens can help treat bladder infections, pneumonia, and infections associated with breastfeeding.
- Dandelions are cultivated as an edible crop and also for medicinal uses.

Even Martha Stewart has come to the defense of this "weed" in a column that speaks of the virtues of dandelions.

"In Russia," Stewart wrote in her newspaper column, "ask Martha," in May 2002, "the plant is known as 'life elixir,' and its leaves are traditionally steamed and served with sour cream and thinly sliced red onion." Dandelions are also favorite fare in Italy and England. "Almost every part of the dandelion can be consumed. Only the dried-out puffball of seeds is inedible."

If you do decide to give the plant a try, be sure to obtain your dandelions from a clean area, free of pesticides and dog droppings. Also, try to buy young greens because the younger the greens are, the less bitter they will be. And yes, the golden weed growing in your backyard is the same variety that you might encounter at a fancy restaurant.

Another dandelion fact, Stewart points out, is that the plant has a valuable function in growing wild. It typically takes hold in decalcified soil, sending its deep roots down to restore minerals to the topsoil. "Wherever you see dandelions turning a green meadow gold," says Stewart, "the earth is being replenished."

It's ironic that the phrase "not in my backyard" (or NIMBY, for short) has come to signify the desire of people living in the suburbs to keep all manner of perceived hazards away from the vicinity of their homes. Yet, it's such suburbanites themselves who are often the worst offenders when it comes to disseminating poisons on their own property. Remember that when you tell your kids to "go out and play in the yard," you should be providing them with a safe haven, not one you've turned into a mini–toxic waste dump just to get rid of some crabgrass or dandelions.

Tips for Keeping Your Lawn Both Attractive and Safe to Play On

- Keep a sharp blade on your lawn mower and never cut off more than one-third of the grass blades at a time. Grass that is not cut too short will grow better roots, be healthier, and do better in drought conditions. Studies at the University of Maryland have shown that by not cutting turf grasses below three inches, you can control crabgrass just as well or better than by using herbicides.
- Don't bag your grass clippings. Clippings contribute to the nutrients of your grass and soil.
- Proper use of mulch is a very effective way to control weeds without chemicals. Good, organic mulches include grass clippings, leaves, and shredded bark. Organic gardeners also use newspaper and grocery bags under the mulch to further block sunlight from weeds. Pulling weeds by hand is a time-honored way to evict them from your garden. You can also use gardening tools, such as a hoe or forked digger.
- Keeping up a large lawn can take up most summer weekends. Why not think about replacing some of your lawn area with ornamental grasses, wildflowers, or other ground coverings. Once they get established, you'll have much less work to do (no mowing or constant watering), and a much more visually appealing landscape. Let's face it: All green and nothing but green is pretty dull.

CONTROLLING HOUSEHOLD PESTS
WITHOUT POISONS

What comes to mind when you think of "pest control"? An exterminating service? A can of bug spray? Why not think about something as simple as fixing small holes in a screen door or not leaving crumbs in the living room instead. Yes, that's pest control. The term is not reserved solely for chemical solutions. Pest control can be, and is, any action you take to make your home environment as unwelcome to pests as possible, be it something as common as vacuuming and cleaning.

Using Common Sense in Place of Chemicals

Pesticides applied inside your home, even ones you can't smell, present a very real risk to your family and may pose far more of a health hazard than the problem they're intended to solve. All too often, in fact, people rush out to buy a can of bug spray or call in an exterminating service without bothering to determine if they even have a real pest infestation to begin with. Simply seeing a roach, a few ants marching across the kitchen floor, or a mosquito that flies in when the screen door is opened does not mean you are being invaded, no matter how many commercials tell you that "if you've seen one, you have a million more."

"The funny thing is, [pesticides] are basically made to kill people, not pests," says Stephen Tvedten, who spent twenty-five years in the "traditional" exterminating industry. "When I was applying chemicals, we never got control; it doesn't work."

What does work, then? According to Tvedten, you can use safe and simple solutions to every possible pest problem, without having to resort to toxic measures. An example is how he handled a situation he encountered several years ago in Ohio, where he was hired to get a school district out of its pesticide rut (see Chapter 4). Tvedten soon discovered that the schools in question had "everything" in the way of pests, both inside and outside. Using no pesticides, insecticides, or rodenticides, Tvedten subsequently managed to make those schools pest-free. His methods, many of which are simply commonsense approaches to avoiding crawling and flying insect problems, are spelled out in detail in his e-book *The Bug Stops Here: How to Safely and Simply Control Most Household Pests Without Harming Yourself or Your Family,* available in its entirety, free of charge, at his Web site (see "Resources" at the end of this chapter).

Part of the reason for the ever-escalating use of synthetic chemicals to "control" pests, he points out, is the self-perpetuating problem that pesticides themselves have caused by creating resistant species. "Anything will have a certain number of survivors," says Tvedten, and those survivors, along with the extermination of their natural predators, is why pesticide use has escalated to unbelievable proportions. "When Rachel Carson wrote *Silent Spring* in 1962, the United States was using around 900,000 pounds of chemical pesticides," he notes. "We now use 4.5 billion pounds."

Recalling his time spent applying "poisons" to people's homes, Tvedten notes that no one follows up on pesticide applications after the fact, the way a building inspector would examine an addition or renovation to your home. "I put poison in your house and no one ever checks," he says. "The pesticide industry is the only business that every year goes up in sales. If this pesticide doesn't work, we will use another, or more, or we'll use them in combination. It does not work." Then, too, what exterminators tell customers is "safe" often turns out to be anything but. "Every chemical that is banned today was yesterday's solution," he points out.

Using quick chemical fixes for insects may only increase your pest problems, as well as polluting your indoor air and spreading a toxic substance around your house. According to Tvedten, it's not that difficult to achieve dramatic results controlling pests without synthetic chemicals, starting with some very simple procedures, such as eliminating their sources of food and water by keeping surfaces clean. "If you feed your pests and water your pests, you might as well give them names, because you've turned them into pets," is how he puts it. He also advises strongly against overkill. Don't try and destroy every ant in your yard, for example, as ants help control fleas and ticks.

Intelligent Pest Management Tips

The following intelligent pest management tips are from Steve Tvedten's e-book *The Bug Stops Here.*

Ants

The best control for ants is cleanliness. Some species of ants are not common inside a structure but appear sporadically, and other types are found inside only under rare or accidental conditions. Be sure to trim all branches that touch or overhang the building and caulk all visible cracks, crevices, and other openings. Make ant barriers with petroleum jelly, Comet, talcum powder, medicated powder, or food-grade diatomaceous earth (DE), a mineral product mined from the fossilized silica shell remains of algae. (Note that if you decide to use talcum powder, check the label first. Some brands still contain asbestos and are therefore carcinogenic for humans.)

Mosquitoes

Noxzema or Ben-Gay applied to the exposed skin of children and adults repels mosquitoes and other pests. First, however, always check for sensitivity to the product before using it.

Dust Mites

The first hurdles to overcome are the beds in your house. That's because a mattress is the resort capital of the dust mites' world. A double bed mattress can hold millions of mites. Pillows and blankets are popular, too. Mattresses and box springs should be encased in zippered, dust-proof covers. Washing bed linens in hot water is crucial. Water hotter than 120 degrees Farenheit can cause accidental scalding, but to kill dust mites, the water must be at least 130 degrees Farenheit. If it's not, use borax and/or Safe Solutions Enzyme Cleaner with Peppermint. Avoid blankets made of wool or down, or routinely wash them in two ounces of Safe Solutions Enzyme Cleaner with Peppermint and/or borax per gallon of water.

Roaches

Create escape-proof barriers with double-sided sticky tape, duct tape with the sticky side up, or petroleum jelly. You can literally trap and remove all the roaches in your home with enough duct tape.

Mix one clove garlic, one onion, one tablespoon of cayenne pepper, and one quart of water. Let the mixture sit for one hour, then strain it, add a tablespoon of liquid soap, and spray it around the house for roach control.

Pests in General

Talcum Powder and/or Medicated Body Powder. Control and/or repel many different kinds of pests in your home by sprinkling around talcum powder or medicated body powder. Talcum powder quickly dries out insects. It repels and controls fire ants and other insect pests and nuisance wildlife. Try using cornstarch in place of talcum powder in vacuums to suffocate vacuumed pests; always use the safest alternative.

Vinegar. Spray weeds and pest plants with vinegar. White vinegar also kills ants. Vinegar attracts wasps, fungus gnats, and fruit flies. Put two inches in a long-necked bottle and add a few drops of liquid soap or enzyme cleaner, and the bugs will crawl in but won't be able to crawl out again.

Lights. Avoid leaving porch lights on all evening to collect a cloud of moths and other insects. Every time the door is opened, the insects swirling around the light are swept into the house.

When designing the lighting around the exterior of a home, don't put light fixtures directly above the doors, especially over the doors to decks or patios that are used a lot in the evening. Use yellow bulbs in yard light fixtures; flies and moths are not as attracted to yellow as they are to ordinary white lightbulbs.

Water. You can control most structure-invading pests simply by controlling the moisture and relative humidity in your home, because water is their most critical survival factor. Do this by installing and properly maintaining dehumidifiers, fans, and air-conditioners, and quickly correcting or repairing all moisture problems.

The Nitty Gritty on Head Lice

If there ever was a case of the "cure" being worse than the problem, it's head lice (often called "cooties" by those under twelve). Despite the rumors surrounding head lice, having them does not mean you're dirty or live in unsanitary conditions. Having head lice is not a disease. You cannot catch head lice from dogs or cats. Lice are not known to transmit infectious agents, and they rarely cause any annoyance other than itching. The real problems posed by head lice are the toxic chemical products you'll be instructed to apply to your child's scalp before he or she will be allowed back in school or day care.

Head lice are parasitic insects that live mainly on the scalp and neck hairs of people, and that are spread by direct contact with a person who has them or with contaminated objects such as clothing and brushes. They shouldn't be confused with body lice, which can carry serious pathogens, such as typhus, and which are infrequently encountered in the United States. Richard J. Pollack, Ph.D., with the Department of Immunology and Infectious Diseases (DIID) Laboratory of Public Health Entomology at the Harvard School of Public Health, believes that the efforts to "seek out" and "quarantine" those suspected of having head lice reflect a misapplication of public-health principles.

This "no nits" policy on head lice is one that Dr. Pollack characterizes as being "imprudent . . . based on misinformation rather than . . . science." The discovery of lice or their eggs on the hair should not cause a child to be sent home or isolated, he maintains. Furthermore, "treatment is not indicated if the infestation is not active." He also points out that children with infections such as colds, by contrast, are rarely banned from school.

The treatments you'll likely be asked to use for head lice are shampoos or rinses containing the pesticide permethrin or pyrethrin, which will not kill the eggs and therefore need to be reapplied as the eggs hatch. Permethrin, a synthetic pyrethroid, is toxic to the nervous system, damages genetic material, affects the reproductive system, stimulates the production of testosterone, and is ranked by the EPA as a possible human carcinogen. Pyrethrins are toxins extracted from species of daisies and can trigger allergic reactions, asthma attacks, and dermatitis, as well as disrupting the nervous system.

Curiously enough, one popular over-the-counter lice treatment containing 1 percent permethrin advises that it is safe for use on infants as young as two months old, while another of the same company's products containing only one-fourth the amount of the pesticide and packaged as a bedding and furniture spray warns on the labeled that it is "not to be used on humans or animals."

If you have used pesticide treatments for lice in the past and found them not to be effective, it probably isn't because you were applying them incorrectly. The discovery of permethrin-resistant lice by researchers from the Harvard School of Public Health explains why more applications (at even higher, prescription-strength concentrations) of permethrin still won't work. A class-action lawsuit in Texas against the manufacturers of several lice treatment products claims that companies are misleading consumers into thinking they have been reinfested or are not using the products correctly when, in fact, lice have become resistant to the chemical.

So, what is a safe treatment? Whoever coined the word "nit-picking" certainly knew, because that's exactly the kind of solution that you can implement without putting your child at risk. Removing the nits (eggs) and lice from the scalp with a fine-tooth nit comb is the safest way to "de-louse." True, the process may be time consuming and tedious, especially when the child has curly hair, but it's both safe and a lot more effective than pouring poison on your child's head. (For curly or coarse hair, it might be easier to pick nits by first wetting the hair or applying a conditioner or oil.)

To do it right, you'll need a bright light and possibly a magnifying glass. Comb through the hair a small section at a time, frequently removing the lice and nits from the comb. Other methods include the application of olive oil to the scalp, which is then wrapped in plastic for several hours (the nits will still need to be removed), and using an enzyme-based preparation, such as Steven Tvedten's nonpesticide enzyme product Lice R Gone, available at his Web site (see "Resources" at the end of this chapter).

Do you need to treat your house or car for lice? No, according to Dr. Pollack; lice and eggs soon die when not on a person. "The chances of a live head louse or egg becoming reunited with a person would seem remote," he says.

What you do need to clean, however, are pillowcases, sheets, pajamas, towels, and even stuffed toys, but not by spraying them with a pesticide. Plain old hot water and soap, as in the washing machine, will do just fine.

For a complete rundown of lice facts and information, see Dr. Pollack's Web page on the subject at www.hsph.harvard.edu/headlice.html#Enzyme.

WHEN WHAT YOU DON'T KNOW CAN HURT YOU

Sometimes, being aware of potential threats to your family's health is your best defense against those very things. Such is the case with toxic mold and chemical sensitivity, either one of which can result in a mind-numbing array of physical and even psychological problems, unless you take steps to keep your family protected.

Toxic Mold: The "Alien" That Lurks in the Damp and the Dark

Anyone who's seen the movie *Ghostbusters* will recall the term that the fearless trio often used following a particularly messy encounter with a house-haunting spook: "I've been slimed." That same expression could be used by hapless homeowners to describe the distinctly unfunny experiences they've had, not with supernatural beings, but with natural ones that seem to have even greater powers to make people sick and literally drive them out of their homes.

The toxic molds that are increasingly being found in residential buildings of all ages and descriptions—from old apartment buildings to brand-new luxury homes—may not fit into the category of harmful synthetic chemicals, but they are another of the pernicious health hazards that our homes can be harboring. Reports of the damage they've done to people's lives have been turning up in many different locales, as well as in the media.

Some molds are considered little more than a nuisance, staining floors, walls, and ceilings and, at worst, causing sinus problems, skin irritations, coughs, and cold symptoms in susceptible individuals. But others, with names like *Stachybotrys* and *Aspergillus*, as well as some types of *Penicillium*, produce airborne spores and mycotoxins that many experts believe are responsible for far more serious health effects. Entering the body via the nose, mouth, or skin, they have been blamed for a whole litany of complaints—among them headaches, dizziness, chronic fatigue, depression, nausea, memory impairment, and bleeding of the nose and lungs—and triggering asthmatic conditions. Toxic mold infestations have even been implicated in cases of infant death.

One five-year-old patient brought in to see Dr. Magaziner had been suffering recurrent fevers and respiratory infections requiring frequent antibiotics and even steroids to control her symptoms. It wasn't until Dr. Magaziner recommended that the child's home be tested for mold, however, that she began to show marked improvement. Several colonies of mold were found in her bedroom, which was adjacent to the bathroom, as well as in the kitchen and family room. Once this particular mold problem was remedied, the girl's fevers and infections were virtually eliminated.

Dr. Magaziner has also treated many other patients who were found to be allergic to mold, and whose symptoms, including chronic headaches, depression, chronic fatigue, and recurrent upper respiratory infections and sinusitis, were alleviated by allergy shots. In such cases, he has found that building up the immune system with nutrients like vitamin C, bioflavonoids, acidophilus, zinc, pantothenic acid, selenium, and vitamin E also plays an important role in eliminating chronic symptoms induced by allergies to mold.

According to one authority on the subject, Dr. Michael Gray of Benson, Arizona, toxic mold spores can lodge deep in the lungs, obstructing and infecting airways, while mycotoxins can attack the brain and suppress the immune system, making victims vulnerable to infection.[5]

While not all scientists are ready to concede that the effects of mold can be that serious, many of the families whose homes have been "haunted" by these creeping and floating fungi have suffered extensive physical distress and financial damage. They tell similar horror stories of having belatedly become aware of the cause of their symptoms, only to discover that cleaning up the problem, which insurance often doesn't cover, can cost many thousands of dollars.

Even celebrities have not been spared. Ed McMahon, for instance, sued his insurer and several other parties for $20 million over an allegedly faulty pipe repair that he claimed caused toxic mold to invade his Beverly Hills mansion. As a result, he charged, he and his wife became seriously ill and his sheepdog died from a respiratory ailment. And Erin Brockovich, the legal activist whose exploits became the subject of a hit movie, nearly lost her $800,000 dream home to hidden mold (and became ill in the process), an experience that caused her to successfully lobby for passage of new mold-protection legislation in California. What produces these toxic organisms is no mystery, however. They tend to grow wherever there are leaks, persistently wet surfaces, or water damage. Thriving best in locales that are damp and dark, they often lurk in basements, under floors, and behind walls—any place where a hidden (or not-so-hidden) source of moisture might exist. Worse yet, mold can spread rather quickly, multiplying at rapid speeds and jumping from room to room.

What's the best way to either prevent or eradicate a toxic mold problem? Here are a few suggestions offered by the EPA:

- Clean up any indoor leaks or spills within twenty-four to forty-eight hours.
- Dry any surfaces or pipes on which condensation may have collected.
- See that the ground outside your home slopes away from the foundation to prevent water from seeping in.
- Make sure roof gutters are kept clean, free of leaves and debris, and in good repair.
- Keep air-conditioning drip pans and drain lines clean and unobstructed.
- Keep the indoor relative humidity below 60 percent (ideally between 30 and 50 percent) by using a dehumidifer if necessary. (The relative humidity can be measured with a small moisture or humidity meter, available at many hardware stores.)
- Run a bathroom fan or keep a window open when showering.
- Fix plumbing leaks as soon as possible.
- Use detergent and water to scrub mold off hard surfaces, and dry thoroughly.
- Throw away moldy items made of absorbent or porous material, such as carpets and ceiling tiles (which should also be checked in schools and offices, since they may become damp

and moldy from water leaks and need to be replaced as soon as possible).

• Do not paint or caulk over moldy surfaces without first cleaning up the mold and drying the surface.

• Consult a restoration specialist if you wish to salvage an item and are unsure how to clean it.

Other tips for discouraging mold growth include circulating air using small electric or ceiling fans; sprinkling borax powder in mold-prone areas like the bottoms of garbage cans; avoiding the use of wallpaper (especially in bathrooms); opening the bathroom window to increase ventilation; leaving a light on in the shower and drying the tub and shower curtain with a small fan; replacing heavy carpeting with throw rugs; not leaving wet items such as towels and washcloths hanging on racks or lying around; and extending your rainspout to carry water farther away from the house.

Poor maintenance and neglected leaks have also made mold a problem in many public schools. So don't be too quick to dismiss your kids' complaints that going to school makes them sick or gives them headaches, as there might very well be an environmental cause that could be doing long-term damage to their health. If you suspect toxic exposure to be the cause, start asking questions; if necessary, investigate the conditions by inspecting the facility yourself, talking to teachers and administrators, and comparing notes with other parents.

Remember, when in doubt, it's better to take your child out, at least until the hazard has been eliminated. And that's often best accomplished by parents and teachers getting together and demanding quick corrective action.

Chemical Sensitivity: Creating a Toxic Overload

It would be bad enough if the effects of environmental poisons were limited to the risk of various types of cancer, damage to vital organs, and neurological ailments. But with the accelerated production and use of synthetic chemicals has come a corresponding increase in a debilitating condition for which limited treatment options are currently available. This condition is multiple chemical sensitivity, or MCS, often referred to simply as chemical sensitivity or chemical injury. Its frequently incapacitating symptoms include blinding headaches, nausea, disorientation, chronic fatigue, memory impairment, brain fog (the inability to think straight), and respiratory problems. All are triggered by coming into contact with the smell of any number of common chemicals, such as household cleaners and detergents, paints, perfumes and fragrances, floor polishes, gasoline, and pesticides (even those drifting from another locale).

MCS is most often believed to result either from a "close encounter" with a highly toxic substance—for instance, fumes from the glue used to install flooring in an improperly ventilated room—or from more prolonged, if less intense, exposure to one or more noxious chemicals. Dr. Rea compares what he calls the "total body load" of accumulated toxic exposures to a rain barrel, with each substance encountered, be it from air pollution, indoor pollution, food pollution, or other sources, filling the barrel up drop by drop until it becomes overloaded and overflows, causing symptoms to manifest themselves. One MCS victim, Australian Diana Crumpler, who chronicled her illness and those of her children in a book entitled *Chemical Crisis* (Scribe Publications, 1994), attributed the condition to the constant and concentrated use of pesticides in the agricultural environment in which she lived.[6]

Victims of mild to moderate MCS often find themselves having to move to places that are relatively free of pollutants and to banish as many common synthetic substances from their immediate environment as possible. Those suffering from more severe cases have had to retreat into total isolation, becoming virtual prisoners in their own homes, unable to tolerate even such conveniences as computers and fax machines—and for that matter, visitors wearing any type of cosmetic, fragrance, or synthetic article of apparel. Others have successfully managed to treat themselves—that is, to lower their total toxic load—by creating a "safe room" in their home. This room is typically free of carpeting; has natural flooring material such as tile, marble, limestone, or hardwood; has its air purified via a HEPA filter; and is devoid of synthetic materials and furnishings.

Conventional medicine has long dismissed or disputed even the existence of such a condition, claiming that its symptoms are psychosomatic, or stress-related. Underlying much of this resistance has been the fear that acknowledging the validity of chemical sensitivity in an increasingly chemical-dependent society would open the door to a vast new area of liability and worker compensation. It thus comes as no surprise that organizations funded by industry, such as the American Council on Science and Health, have attempted to portray those who suffer from the affliction as hypochondriacs and therapies for it as "junk science."

In recent years, however, chemical sensitivity as an environmentally triggered illness has come to be more and more recognized as a legitimate condition, to which the field of environmental medicine has devoted an increasing amount of attention. This has largely been the result of a steadily growing number of cases. Individuals displaying classic symptoms of MCS have included workers at the headquarters of the EPA, suffering an apparent response to "sick-building syndrome," or a building filled with toxic fumes—and many Desert Storm veterans suffering from so-called Gulf War syndrome.[7] Also affected have been some mainstream medical practitioners themselves, who developed symptoms while working at hospitals where chemical cleaning solutions and other toxic substances were in constant use.

One reason why conventional medicine has tended to dismiss chemical sensitivity is that it does not conform to the clinical patterns of the standard allergic response mechanism. But authorities on the subject have seen evidence that exposure to toxic substances may cause adverse chemical changes to occur in the brains of susceptible individuals, a reaction that allergists simply are not equipped to detect or diagnose. According to Dr. Claudia S. Miller, a specialist in environmental and occupational medicine at the University of Texas Health Science Center at San Antonio who has spent many years researching the condition, environmental chemicals are capable of disrupting the neurochemistry of the brain's limbic area, a phenomenon seen in animals that she refers to as "olfactory-limbic sensitization." The fact that this area of the brain regulates so many bodily systems, she observes, may explain why MCS has so many different symptoms.[8]

To help deal with this ever-expanding epidemic of environmental illness, a number of alternative medical centers and clinics have sprung up in various parts of the country, offering procedures such as avoidance therapy, sauna detoxification, and treatments aimed at boosting the immune system. These treatments are more or less effective depending, as in other illnesses, on how far the condition has progressed.

A far better method of protecting yourself and your family from the life-altering (and sometimes life-threatening) manifestations of chemical sensitivity, however, is to keep the level of toxic chemicals in your own "rain barrel" as low as possible. You might not be able to avoid them all, but the choices you make can help keep your family's immediate environment relatively free of certain outdoor and indoor pollutants, such as pesticides, air fresheners, varnishes, and toxic glues. You can, for instance, take such preventive steps as using natural pest control methods, cleaning your home with harmless compounds, and using less toxic paints (those with low odor formulations). In addition, when the time comes to replace your carpeting, you can opt for hardwood floors instead (using less volatile glues).

Glues, paints, cleaning agents, and other chemical substances that smell really noxious, as well as places that have an overwhelming chemical odor (such as a hotel or office that has recently installed new carpeting), should be avoided whenever possible. Windows should also be kept open as much as possible, since ventilation is one of the best ways to reduce the level of chemical substances in the air inside a building. Chemicals that smell really bad are giving you a message: Don't just put up with it and treat it as an annoyance. Follow your nose—hopefully out the door into some fresh air!

After nearly two decades of treating hundreds of patients with varying degrees of chemical sensitivity, Dr. Magaziner has found that evaluating each patient's individual biochemistry is essential. Many of these individuals have defective detoxification pathways—that is, their liver's ability to rid the body of toxins is often sluggish or even impaired. He has also noted that trace mineral imbalances are not uncommon in people with MCS, who frequently have a deficiency of magnesium, zinc, or selenium.

Recently, more victims of MCS have also been found to have excessive levels of toxic metals such as lead, cadmium, mercury, arsenic, nickel, or tin, since these substances are becoming more pervasive in our air, water, and food supply (see Chapter 6). And once again, people with MCS may not have the ability to effectively excrete these heavy metals. Dr. Magaziner has also found evidence that people with MCS may have a specific DNA pattern that increases susceptibility to developing this syndrome. Sophisticated laboratory testing is now available to identify whether or not a deletion or defect in your genetic material may make you prone to MCS.

Over the years, Dr. Magaziner has had increased success in treating MCS through improving the immune response with organic whole foods, administering nutritional supplements both orally and intravenously, treating concurrent underlying infections with natural agents, using oxygen therapy and allergy desensitization, and removing toxic metals from the body. Another therapy that has proven highly effective is sauna detoxification, which induces the "sweating out" of chemicals stored in the liver and other tissues. The purpose of all such treatments is to lower the body's total load of poisons to the point where the "rain barrel" is no longer full. This gives the body a chance to heal so that the symptoms eventually disappear.

The bottom line: If you or a member of your family is suffering symptoms of chemical sensitivity, seek out a physician who understands the intricacies of the condition, rather than a conventional practitioner, who is apt to be unfamiliar with its causes and treatments. In addition, make sure to get a thorough biochemical, nutritional, and allergy evaluation. Doctors who are members of the American Academy of Environmental Medicine or the American College for the Advancement of Medicine are often highly trained in diagnosing and treating MCS. (See "Resources" at the end of this chapter.)

You may not be able to control much of what goes on in the outside world, but as noted at the start of this book, your home is indeed your castle when it comes to what, as well as whom, you allow inside. It's the one place where you call the shots and can set up the kind of nontoxic environment that will help your kids develop into healthier adults. And who knows—you may even inspire those who visit your home to do likewise, until eventually the idea of eliminating household poisons catches on with a majority of families. Then, perhaps, the outside world, too, will start to become a less toxic place for children to play and grow up in.

RESOURCES

Alternatives to Pesticides

The Best Control
Web site: www.thebestcontrol.com
   The Web site of Steve Tvedten, the best source for pesticide-free alternatives to bug control. Offers Tvedten's 84-page book *The Bug Stops Here*, which can be printed out for free.

Beyond Pesticides: National Coalition Against the Misuse of Pesticides (NCAMP)
Web site: www.beyondpesticides.org
   The Web site of NCAMP, based in Washington, DC, which has been providing information to the public about pesticides

and their alternatives since 1981. Its "Safety Source for Pest Management" section, linked off the home page, is an extensive directory and resource containing information on nontoxic pest management and more.

Bio-Integral Resource Center (BIRC)
Web site: www.birc.org
    The Web site of BIRC, which specializes in finding nontoxic and least-toxic integrated pest management (IPM) solutions.

Northwest Coalition for Alternatives to Pesticides (NCAP)
Web site: www.pesticide.org
    The Web site of NCAP, based in Eugene, Oregon, which works to advance nontoxic solutions to pest problems.

Pesticide Action Network North America (PANNA)
Web site: www.panna.org
    The Web site of PANNA, based in San Francisco, which has been campaigning since 1982 to replace pesticides with environmentally safe alternatives. Offers plenty of nonchemical and low-toxicity solutions to most pest problems.

Safe Solutions
Web site: www.safesolutionsinc.com
    Sells Steve Tvedten's enzyme solutions, natural weed killer, and nonpesticide head lice treatment.

Alternatives to Toxic Household Products

Children's Health Environmental Coalition (CHEC)
Web site: www.checnet.org
    Articles, advice, and tips on reducing risks for infants and children, as well as prenatal exposures.

A Consumer Guide to Safer Alternatives to Hazardous Household Products

Web site: http://es.epa.gov/new/contacts/newsltrs/shopping.html
An extensive listing of substitutes for commonly used hazardous household products from the EPA's Enviroene Web site.

Less Lawn
Web site: www.lesslawn.com
Techniques, designs, options, and resources for anyone looking for alternatives to traditional turf lawn.

Seventh Generation
Web site: www.seventhgeneration.com
Sells cleaning products that contain nontoxic, phosphate-free, and biodegradable ingredients and that are not tested on animals.

Physician Referrals

American Academy of Environmental Medicine (AAEM)
7701 East Kellogg
Suite 625
Wichita, KS 67207
Telephone: 316-684-5500
Web site: www.aaem.com
Referrals to nutritionally oriented physicians.

American College for Advancement in Medicine (ACAM)
23121 Verdugo Drive
Suite 204
Laguna Hills, CA 92653
Telephone: 800-532-3688
Web site: www.acam.org
Referrals to nutritionally oriented physicians.

❁ **6** ❁

Heavy Metals: No Brainers

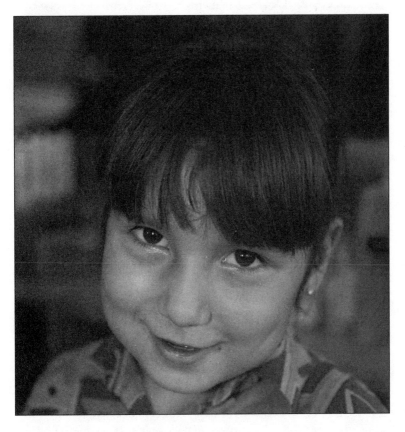

"Lead poisoning destroys dreams."
—Whitlynn Battle, founder, Mothers' Environmental
Coalition of Alabama

WHAT YOU'LL FIND IN THIS CHAPTER

The threat that lead poisoning poses to America's children is considered by many to be the country's number-one health concern. Today, we are paying the price for allowing paint with a high content of this brain-damaging metal to be used for so many years, as the interiors and exteriors of numerous homes shed their toxic skins, leaving residues of hazardous chips and dust for youngsters to ingest. The result has been a marked decline in many a child's capacity to learn, as well as an increase in behavioral problems and in other serious effects on the physical and emotional health of numerous children. These problems are now being tackled by dedicated community groups with the help of federal lead-abatement programs. Other efforts to "get the lead out" include a growing number of lawsuits aimed at the paint companies, which have been accused of knowing of lead's hazards even as they continued to use it in their products. Children are inadvertently exposed to lead in other ways as well, such as through their parents' occupations and hobbies.

Another heavy metal, mercury, is also a neurotoxic nightmare. If ever there was a substance that should be scrupulously avoided by both children and adults, mercury is it. Yet this potentially deadly metal, with its toxic fumes and mind-destroying propensity, is something with which we all may too easily come into contact—in such ordinary sources as dental fillings, thermometers, batteries, fluorescent lights, and coal-burning power plants. Mercury poisoning, however, isn't always apparent to medical professionals and may be diagnosed as some other condition—and left untreated—unless a doctor knows what to look for. The use of mercury as a preservative in many childhood vaccines is also believed by many people to have caused their children to become autistic after receiving multiple immunizations at one time. This is one of several purported links between vaccinations and the sharp rise in the cases of autism. While that connection is strongly denied by the American Medical Association and others representing the medical profession, hearings chaired by an influential congressman who alleges that his grandson is among the affected children were followed by an FDA call for mercury to be removed from vaccine formulas. Existing stocks, however, remain in use, even as lawyers have begun suing the vaccine manufacturers on behalf of the parents of the children they claim were damaged by mercury in immunizations.

Things You Can Do Now!

- Have your children's blood checked to determine its lead content. (Urine and stool samples may also reveal the presence of high lead levels.)
- If your child is found to have higher-than-normal lead levels, take steps to determine the source, whether it be lead dust from old paint in your home or some other locale, the pipes that deliver your tap water, or some other means of exposure.
- If your home was built prior to 1978, have it tested for lead, especially if you have young children or are expecting a child. If high levels are detected in existing paint, have the paint removed by a lead-abatement professional.
- Avoid other possible lead hazards by discarding old miniblinds and making sure that any calcium supplements given to your child are labeled as being "lead-free."
- Make a point of telling your dentist that you don't want amalgam fillings, which contain mercury, in your child's mouth (or your own).
- If you still have a mercury thermometer, replace it immediately with a nontoxic variety, and make sure to properly dispose of the old one via your community's hazardous waste–collection program.

Imagine, if you will, living in a country where a large part of the citizenry is suffering from some degree of brain damage. It's a frightening prospect, indeed, but one that could very well characterize the state of American society in the not-too-distant future, thanks to our having too long allowed industry to have a free hand in the manufacture of products containing such heavy metals as lead and mercury. To be sure, some restrictive measures have been belatedly placed on the use of these hazardous materials, but not before the stage was set for a great deal of potential damage from them. That's why it's imperative that responsible parents be aware of the still existing dangers and take whatever steps are necessary to shield their kids from the damage that heavy metals can inflict on their minds and potentials.

LEAD'S TOXIC LEGACY AND ITS THREAT TO OUR FUTURE

In 1996, when Destiny Askew was only two years old, she lived up to her name by becoming the catalyst for a movement that would help assure many other children in Alabama of—quite literally—a brighter future. It was while waiting at the office of Destiny's pediatrician that her mother, Lynn, picked up a copy of *Good Housekeeping* magazine and read an article about childhood lead poisoning.

"We fit all of the criteria for the high-risk groups," said Lynn, who lives in Birmingham. "So when we saw the doctor, I asked about Destiny's lead levels. I assumed that she had been tested."

The pediatrician hadn't tested Destiny, nor did she believe it was required. "She told me that she had been practicing medicine for over 20 years, and she had never found it necessary to test a child for lead poisoning before," said Lynn. But while insisting that lead poisoning was not a problem in Birmingham, but only in large Northeastern cities, the doctor finally gave in to Lynn and did the simple—and relatively inexpensive—test.

The lead levels in Destiny's blood were low by state standards; at 10 micrograms per deciliter (ug/dl), they didn't even begin to meet the legal criteria for lead poisoning. But it was enough to get Lynn's attention.

"The doctor said not to worry, they would test her again in three months," Lynn recalls. "But everything I had read led me to believe that in three months things were probably going to be the same or worse. The doctor didn't tell me a thing about lead poisoning, just 'don't worry, it will probably go away.' "

Calling the local health department for assistance, Lynn learned that to meet the legal standard for lead poisoning in Alabama, a blood level of at least 17 ug/dl, no matter what your age, is necessary. Lynn then had her house tested for lead, but the finding was negative, as was the finding for her mother's house. Locating no source of paint contamination, the most common cause of elevated lead levels, Lynn started searching the Internet, where she first found out about the "calcium connection." Being lactose intolerant, as many African-American children are, Destiny had been taking a calcium supplement for about a year after breaking her leg. Ironically, as her mother discovered, although a high-calcium diet is helpful in reducing lead levels, it was the calcium supplement Destiny was taking that was actually causing her lead exposure. That's because many calcium supplements are contaminated with lead from pollution. Having discovered this information, Lynn immediately took Destiny off the supplement, and within ninety days, the girl's lead level fell from 10 ug/dl to 2 ug/dl. "I had been dosing my child with lead every day," she says.

Lynn's involvement could have stopped right there; the mystery had been solved, and Destiny's lead level had dropped substantially. But during a call for information she made to the National Safety Council in Washington, DC, she was told that although there was money available for a nonprofit organization dealing with lead education in the state of Alabama, nobody "willing to take it" could be found.

"I started thinking, who could take this money? Then I got an idea," says Lynn. Despite having "no notion of what I was doing," she managed to turn that idea into an organization called Citizens' Lead Education and Poisoning Prevention, and eventually into another called the Mothers' Environmental Coalition of Alabama. As hands-on coordinator of the campaign as well as its founder, Lynn has since dedicated herself to personally guiding the families of lead-poisoning victims through the thicket of bureaucracy to a relatively lead-free environment, including making arrangements for them to be relocated if necessary and to receive whatever aid money is available. Working for no salary, she has also spearheaded a drive to have blood tests administered to children in schools and neighborhoods where the risks of lead exposure are highest.

"Lead poisoning doesn't leave any outward symptoms; by the time a parent finds out there's a big problem, it's too late," cautions Lynn. "If your child's blood lead level is 5 or 6 or 7 mg/dl, for example, you don't know if that number is on the way up, or on the way down."

There are other possible reasons for concern, even if a child's blood lead level is not considered all that significant. Results of research done in 2001 at the Children's Hospital Medical Center in Cincinnati indicate that even relatively low levels of lead may still adversely affect reading and math scores.[1] While average blood lead levels in American children have declined since the 1970s, Dr. Bruce Lanphear, who did the Children's Hospital study, believes that childhood lead exposure is "still a major public health crisis in the U.S." The Alliance to End Childhood Lead Poisoning goes even further, claiming that "despite significant progress in reducing lead poisoning, it remains the number one environmental health hazard facing American children."

But then, "there is no magic number for lead poisoning," says Dr. Lanphear. "The science shows that any lead exposure hurts fetuses and young children."

Lead Poisoning: Any Child Is a Potential Victim

Lead is a systemic poison for people of all ages, with those most vulnerable being infants, toddlers, and pregnant women. In fact, while the average adult absorbs 10 to 15 percent of the lead that reaches the digestive tract, according to the FDA, young children and pregnant women absorb much more—as much as 50 percent—with the rate even higher for people suffering from calcium deficiencies, a frequent problem among poor and inner-city children. This heavy metal can affect a child's rapidly developing brain, causing learning disabilities and behavioral problems. At very high levels, lead poisoning can be fatal. Lead can also cross the placenta and adversely affect the developing fetus.

"The old stereotype is that children only got lead poisoning by eating paint chips, and these were children with inattentive parents," notes Tom Matte, a medical epidemiologist and physician with the CDC's National Center for Environmental Health. But lead ingestion, he points out, goes hand in hand (or actually, hand in mouth) with being a child. "Mouthing behavior is normal. Their hand, any object in fact, goes in their mouth. It's the first thing a very young child does to check something out." And lead dust, which can contaminate both the inside and the outside of a home, is easily ingested that way. "Lead is a preventable cause of keeping children from reaching their full potential," says Matte.

Lead can certainly impact greatly on a school-age child's ability to learn. In fact, research has shown that the level of lead in the teeth of young children may be an accurate predictor of how well they will perform academically in middle school and high school. When scientists measured the lead levels in the baby teeth of six- and seven-year-olds (after the teeth fell out), they found that those children with the highest levels were more likely to have learning problems in school, have greater absenteeism, and engage in more antisocial behavior. In fact, those with the highest levels were less likely to complete high school than those with the lowest levels of lead in their teeth.

Lead prevention starts with investigation of the environment in which children spend time, be it their own home, their grandparents' home, or the day-care facility. Prevention is the best way to protect a child against lead poisoning. Don Ryan, executive director of the Alliance to End Childhood Lead Poisoning, perhaps put it best when he said that children ought not to be "lead detectors."

"Truly protecting U.S. children from lead poisoning requires us to start testing houses, as well as children," Ryan maintains, an opinion supported by the fact that an estimated 40 percent of American homes contain lead paint, according to the U.S. Department of Housing and Urban Development. The prevalence of the problem, in fact, has prompted some three dozen municipal, state, and county governments, including the city of Chicago, to file litigation aimed at forcing paint companies, which are alleged to have concealed the hazards of lead-based paint from the public, to be held responsible for cleaning it up.

Since young children are especially sensitive to the effects of lead, assessing your child's environment for possible lead exposures is of vital importance. (You should take equal measures if you are pregnant.) According to the CDC, the main risk factor for lead exposure comes from the lead paint in older housing. By that we mean any home or building that was built prior to 1978 and especially before 1950. Lead-based paints were commonly used until the late 1970s, both on the interiors and exteriors of homes and buildings and on furniture. Paint chips are not the only hazard for which to look. Lead paint contaminates dust, which can be in the air, on the floor, and on windowsills, and is easily ingested by children while putting objects and hands in their mouths.

Experts emphasize that you should not attempt to rid your home of lead paint yourself. In fact, some of the worst exposures to lead occur during paint stripping and renovations. Lead removal is definitely something best left to professionals; trying to do it yourself can actually make the problem far worse.

ARE YOU PLANNING TO BUY OR RENT A HOME BUILT BEFORE 1978?

Federal law requires that individuals receive certain information before renting or buying pre-1978 housing. The residential lead-based paint disclosure program says in part:

- A landlord has to disclose known information on lead-based paint and lead-based paint hazards in the home before the lease takes effect. The leases must include a disclosure form about lead-based paint.
- A seller has to disclose known information on lead-based paint and lead-based paint hazards in the home before selling it. The sales contract must include a disclosure form about lead-based paint. The buyer has up to ten days to check for lead hazards.

Source: U.S. Environmental Protection Agency.

The Risks of Lead Exposure to the Unborn

While the toxic effects of lead on infants and toddlers are the primary focus of both local and federal government agencies, lead also impacts the fetus in very significant ways. A pregnant woman's exposure to lead can increase her risk of premature delivery, as well as result in lower birth weight and impairment of the baby's mental development.[2] Those effects on the developing fetus have been noted at maternal blood lead levels of 10 to 15 ug/dl, although it is not known if lower levels can have similar toxic effects.[3] Women whose work exposes them to high levels of lead also have a greater chance of spontaneous abortion, and most importantly, the lowest blood level that could put a woman at risk has not yet been established.[4] Again, you don't have to be constantly exposed—either an acute exposure (a significant dose on one or more occasions) or chronic (over a long period of time) low-dose exposure can jeopardize your pregnancy.

Lead can adversely affect the reproductive process in men as well. Studies on men who work with lead have shown a considerable lowering of sperm count, which also can result from either an acute exposure or chronic low-dose exposures.

A Link Between Lead Poisoning and Fluoridated Water?

As discussed in Chapter 1, fluoride is a toxic substance of dubious value in reducing cavities. Another reason to eliminate its use in public water supplies comes from the results of a study involving 280,000 Massachusetts children done by Professors Roger D. Masters and Myron J. Coplan, and published in the *International Journal of Environmental Studies* in 1999. The researchers found that those living in communities whose water had been treated with what is by far the most common source of fluoride, silicofluorides (SiFs), had significantly higher blood lead levels. Other studies have corroborated these results, which tend to support

Masters's theory that SiFs act to increase the cellular uptake of lead.

Masters, a Dartmouth College research professor, says that if further studies confirm their findings, "[SiFs] may well be the worst environmental poison since leaded gasoline."

A Checklist for Lead Risk

You may think you've created a lead-free environment for your children, but some factors may have "slipped through the cracks." Here's a list of six possible lead hazard situations you may have overlooked:

1. Does your child spend any time in a structure built before 1978 (including the home of a friend, grandparents, or sitter, as well as a day-care or preschool facility)?
2. Does your child spend any time in a structure built before 1978 that has been renovated or is undergoing renovations? That's a possible red flag, as renovations done unprofessionally, or without regard to lead hazards, might well make the problem worse.
3. Do you, or does anyone else who lives with your child, engage in work or hobbies that expose them to lead? If so, any clothing worn during the work should be changed before returning home and laundered separately from your child's clothing. Such occupations include:

- Automobile repair, including painting and especially battery work
- Any custodial or maintenance work
- Hair dressing (many hair dyes contain lead)
- Contracting and/or remodeling work
- Farm work (agricultural soil may contain high levels of lead due to the use of leaded fuel in farm machinery over a period of many decades)

- Pottery making or glass blowing (lead is found in many pottery glazes)

4. Does your home have old pipes? Lead in pipes can contaminate drinking and cooking water. Another source in pipes is lead solder, which wasn't banned until the late 1980s. To flush any possible lead out before using your water, simply let the cold water run for about a minute every morning. Never cook with hot water from the faucet, and *never use hot water from the faucet to make infant formula.* If you do have any lead in your pipes, more of it will leach out when using hot water. Again, as discussed in Chapter 3, think about using water filtered through reverse osmosis, which removes lead.

5. Do your children, or anyone who lives with them, spend any time at a shooting range? (See "Guns: A Toxic Threat as Well" on page 184.)

6. What industries are in your environment? Active smelters and battery-recycling plants release lead into the atmosphere, which in turn creates lead-contaminated dust.

Other Possible Sources of Lead Exposure at Home

Even if your home and other places your child visits are free of lead paint, there are still various ways by which lead can be inadvertently brought into your house.

Older Vinyl Miniblinds

In the summer of 1996, the U.S. Consumer Product Safety Commission (CPSC) reported that 25 million foreign-made miniblinds containing lead were being imported into the United States each year. When sunlight hits vinyl containing lead, it causes the vinyl to degrade and produce lead dust. (Dusting such blinds doesn't help—the dust will just contaminate the air, windowsills,

GUNS: A TOXIC THREAT AS WELL

Just when you thought there couldn't be any more bad things to say about mixing kids and guns comes a warning from the Violence Policy Center (VPC) in Washington, DC, about lead pollution from both indoor and outdoor shooting ranges.

The VPC reports in its 2001 study "Poisonous Pastime" that it's been known since the 1970s that outdoor shooting ranges are major sources of environmental lead pollution and that indoor shooting ranges can cause lead poisoning in people who use them.

Lead contamination from these sources can be so significant that a day-care center in Florida had to close down due to lead-contaminated air that was vented into its playground area from a neighboring shooting range.[5]

The VPC warns that secondary lead poisoning can occur when clothing contaminated at the range carries lead dust home. Contamination can also occur by washing a child's clothing with items containing lead dust.

Any child who has had direct or indirect exposure to a shooting range should have his or her blood lead levels tested immediately. Furthermore, no child should ever be allowed in a shooting range or be exposed to ammunition reloading, the VPC emphasizes.

and floor.) The Window Covering Manufacturers Association has since reached a voluntary agreement with the CPSC to replace the lead used in the manufacturing process with tin. Newer blinds produced in this manner should bear a sticker stating that no lead has been added, and by this time, according to the CPSC, the chances of any lead-containing miniblinds still being on the market are slim.

The fact that lead-containing miniblinds are no longer being sold, however, doesn't mean they're extinct. If you have any vinyl miniblinds in your home that were manufactured before 1997, and you have young children in that home, you should replace the blinds immediately. If you're not sure how old your miniblinds are, it's best to be on the safe side and get new ones.

Remember one of the primary rules of maintaining a nontoxic home: When in doubt, throw it out.

Candles with Wicks Containing Lead

Burning candles with lead-containing wicks will emit lead in the air and also deposit lead onto surfaces in the room. You cannot tell just by looking at a candle if its wick has a lead core or not. In the mid-1970s, the U.S. candle industry stopped using lead-cored wicks; however, these wicks mysteriously reappeared on the market a short time later.[6] The CPSC in 2002 issued a proposed rule that, if passed, would ban candles with wicks that contain more than 0.06 percent lead. In the meantime, the U.S. candle industry states that it has voluntarily eliminated lead wicks.

Imports, however, can still pose a hazard unless a mandatory rule is established and goes into full effect. A few countries have already taken steps, though. Australia and New Zealand have put provisional bans on candles with lead-containing wicks, and Denmark banned a number of candle products containing lead in 2000.

Calcium Supplements

After a good deal of publicity was given to a 1993 study published in the *American Journal of Public Health* that found a quarter of some seventy calcium supplements tested exceeded the FDA's lead limits, manufacturers of such supplements promised to get the lead out. However, a subsequent study done in 2001 found substantial levels of lead still remaining in both natural and refined calcium supplements.[7] "Natural" calcium supplements include those made of oyster shells and bone meal. However, the study detected lead in four out of seven natural products, as well as in four out of fourteen refined ones.[8]

As Lynn Battle found out, taking such supplements can cause your child's lead blood levels to rise. Pregnant women should also avoid calcium supplements containing lead. Look for calcium supplements that are labeled "lead-free," or ask the manufacturer if assays are available indicating that the product is lead-free.

Bright and Colorful Dishware

Lead used to brighten the color and sheen of pottery can leach into the food you're serving, especially acidic foods such as tomato sauce and orange juice. Since 1971, the FDA has taken steps to regulate the amount of lead allowed in ceramic ware, with the strictest rules applying to mugs used for serving coffee and tea. While such restrictions are designed to provide a "reasonable margin of protection," they're no guarantee that pottery will be lead-free, particularly with all the dishware available from abroad. It's therefore up to you to follow some basic precautions, such as avoiding the use of extremely decorative dishes for serving food, not storing fruit juices in ceramic or crystal containers, limiting the use of antique or collectible housewares to special occasions, and avoiding the use of ceramic mugs if you're pregnant. You can have your dishes tested for lead, which is really the only way to know for sure.

Protecting Against Lead Exposure

If you suspect that your house has lead hazards, you can take some immediate steps to reduce your family's risk. The following tips are courtesy of the EPA:

- If you rent, notify your landlord of peeling or chipping paint.
- Clean up paint chips immediately.
- Clean floors, window frames, windowsills, and other surfaces weekly. Use a mop, sponge, or paper towel with warm water and a general all-purpose cleaner (we suggest using a mild, nontoxic soap).
- Thoroughly rinse sponges and mop heads after cleaning dirty or dusty areas.

How Many People Does It Take to Dispose of a Lightbulb?

Fluorescent light fixtures, commonly found in offices and schools (and sometimes in kitchens and bathrooms, too) contain small amounts of mercury, which can be released into the air if they break. Mercury is also contained in the new "energy saver" bulbs that are used in place of standard incandescent bulbs. If we want to avoid exposure to mercury vapors and also be more "green," just how do we throw away these bulbs?

We decided to call our local recycling center and ask. We posed our question to three different people dealing with garbage pickup and recycling. Each one told us to just "throw it in the trash," as they do. When we asked if that wouldn't be bad for the environment, as these bulbs contain mercury vapor, they said they weren't aware of that fact. A company that deals in hazardous waste removal gave us even worse advice: "Crush them and put them in with your regular trash."

"But wouldn't that release mercury?" we asked.

"Yes, but that's what we do here."

Considering that fifty teachers and students at a middle school in Alabama were taken to a hospital with skin blisters and red, burning, and swollen eyes after a mercury-containing light fixture shattered, we didn't think that was such a good idea.

So, what should you do? The most logical advice we found comes from the State of Massachusetts Department of Environmental Protection. Its Web page says to try and not throw such fixtures away in the garbage, but rather to find out when your community has a hazardous waste pickup day and bring them in. Your local public works department should have details about when this event is held in your community. To read the article, "Fluorescent Lamp Management for Consumers," on the State of Massachusetts' Web page, go to www.state.ma.us/dep/files/lamps.htm.

And if you save up your used fixtures for such occasions, put them in a place where they are not likely to be broken, and definitely keep them away from toddlers.

- Wash children's hands often, especially before they eat and before naptime and bedtime.
- Keep play areas clean. Wash bottles, pacifiers, toys, and stuffed animals regularly.
- Keep children from chewing windowsills and other painted surfaces.
- Have everyone who enters your home first clean or remove his or her shoes to avoid tracking in lead from soil.
- Make sure your children eat nutritious foods high in iron and calcium, such as spinach and dairy products. Children with good diets absorb less lead.

In addition to day-to-day cleaning and good nutrition, the EPA recommends the following:

- Temporarily reduce any lead hazards in your home by taking actions such as repairing damaged painted surfaces and planting grass over soil with high lead levels. These actions, called "interim controls," are not permanent solutions and will need ongoing attention.
- To permanently remove lead hazards, hire a certified lead "abatement" contractor. Abatement methods include removing, sealing, or enclosing lead-based paint with special materials. Just painting over the hazard with regular paint is not enough.
- Always hire a person with special training to correct lead problems—someone who knows how to do this work safely and has the proper equipment to clean up thoroughly. Certified contractors will employ qualified workers and follow strict safety rules set by the state or federal government.
- Contact the National Lead Information Center (NLIC) for help with locating certified contractors in your area and to see if financial assistance is available.

Leaded Gasoline: What Can Happen When Industry Dictates Policy

Between 1945 and 1971, the period of greatest leaded gasoline use, it's estimated that up to 275,000 tons of lead dust were spit out of the exhaust pipes of American cars each year.[9] Such brain-damaging toxic dust, created by the use of leaded gasoline, coated the American landscape. How did the government let this happen? Didn't we know the dangers of lead back then?

The toxicity of lead, suspected, in part, to be responsible for the fall of Rome (the Romans constructed astounding aqueducts to bring water from the mountains, which was carried to the people by lead pipes within the city), was described back in 1786 in a letter from Benjamin Franklin to a friend. In Franklin's boyhood Boston, rum distilleries were prohibited from using lead parts, which contaminated the spirits, causing paralysis in people. By the 1820s, lead's poisonous qualities were well established.

But in the early 1920s, it seemed that an opportunity for great profits using lead had "knocked," in a perverse kind of way, for three giant companies. Looking for ways to beat Ford's Model T, General Motors (GM) decided that the automobile of the future needed to be more than "basic transportation," something that was both powerful and stylish. GM developed the high-compression engine, which provided greater horsepower but didn't burn regular gasoline well; it produced a "knock." GM chemists solved that annoyance, finding that tetraethyl lead formulated in gasoline stopped the engine knock, and on February 1, 1923, the first leaded gasoline went on sale in Dayton, Ohio.

Produced by what was called the Ethyl Corporation (an alliance of GM, Standard Oil of New Jersey, and DuPont), its manufacture was disastrous from the start. Workers making the fuel in New Jersey suffered tremors, hallucinations, and other serious effects of brain and nerve damage, resulting in five deaths and several workers being committed to insane asylums. Press reports of what was going on in the plants where the lead fuel was being manufactured (DuPont's New Jersey plant was dubbed "The

House of Butterflies," as workers there were experiencing hallucinations of insects) got public health officials involved. After all, if
the people manufacturing leaded gasoline were falling ill at such
a fast rate, what were the risks of spewing this gasoline into the
atmosphere along with automobile exhaust?

In May 1925, the U.S. Public Health Service called a conference on leaded gasoline, and Standard Oil, in an apparent public
relations effort, suspended sales of the product. The conferees,
which included scientists and chemists from industry, academia,
and the government, jointly agreed that the fine lead dust emitted
by the cars using this new gasoline was a cumulative, brain-
damaging poison. But what would be the result of spewing it out
of the rear end of automobiles? No one could say with absolute
certainty—after all, this had never been done before.

Those not affiliated with industry called for caution; Harvard
professor and lead expert Dr. Alice Hamilton was quoted as saying, "This new industrial hazard should not be put into general use
. . . until we have adequate and full information assuring us that
we are not introducing another health hazard into our daily lives."

Industry, however, in a manner remarkably similar to the way
it has promoted the use of toxic pesticides and other chemicals,
urged that the new technology forge ahead, despite all that was
known about lead or suspected might be the consequences of its
use in gasoline. Scientific conjecture, it was argued, shouldn't
stop progress without absolute proof that the effects would be
detrimental.

As a representative of the Ethyl Corporation put it at the 1925
conference, "Our continued development of motor fuels is essential in our civilization . . . [W]e have this apparent gift of God . . .
of tetraethyl lead."

When the May conference ended, all the parties agreed that
further study was needed, and so, for the rest of 1925, the ap-
pointed committee surveyed mechanics and others exposed to the
new lead gas in Ohio. Its conclusion was rosy for the Ethyl Corporation: "There are at present no good grounds for prohibiting
the use of ethyl gasoline." By June 1926, leaded gasoline was back

on the market, and Ethyl continued to make and sell it until Congress outlawed it in 1989.[10]

As journalist Peter Montague points out in his comprehensive article about lead gasoline's tainted past, "The History of Precaution," published in 1997 in the e-zine *Rachel's Environment and Health Weekly*: "The 'facts' could not include any poisonings until such poisoning had already occurred (until they occurred, they would be nothing more than speculative 'fears' or 'opinions') . . . Today the language is slightly different; we hear calls for policy based on 'sound science' (not on 'facts') but it is the same argument."

Getting the Lead Out

If you have any reason to think you might have a problem in regard to lead, there are methods for finding out one way or another. Here are some suggestions for implementing them.

GETTING THE LEAD OUT OF YOUR NEIGHBORHOOD

Want to tackle the problem of preventing lead paint poisoning in your neighborhood or community? The U.S. Department of Housing and Urban Development (HUD) has funds in reserve for states and cities to assist with lead abatement, but many locales still aren't taking advantage of the program. For information on what's being done by your state or city to make use of that money, contact your nearest HUD office.

Testing Lead Levels

Should all young children have their blood lead levels checked? Even if you don't fit into any of the high-risk categories, it's the only real way to know if your child has been exposed to lead. The test is simple and should be done every year until age six. Lynn Battle believes it should be a "parent's choice" to test, not a decision determined by insurance companies or doctors.

Although a blood test is the most common method used by pediatricians to diagnose lead toxicity, it may not be the preferred procedure. Dr. Magaziner and other physicians have found that high levels of lead can often be detected in the urine or stool even when the blood levels are within the normal range. With chronic, low-level exposure, lead will typically be taken up and stored in the tissues, with little actually circulating in the blood.

In Dr. Magaziner's experience, some children excrete lead (and often other toxic metals) through the kidneys, and it can therefore be found in the urine. In other children, it passes through the gastrointestinal tract and can be recovered in the stool. The point is that lead can be hidden in the body, and the fact that there may not be high levels detected in the blood doesn't mean that it's not there.

For instance, one of Dr. Magaziner's patients, four-year-old Matthew, was diagnosed with ADD and developmental delay, only to be found to have toxic levels of lead upon stool and urine assessment, even though his blood tested normal. He was treated for lead poisoning with a chelating agent (a substance that strongly binds with toxic metals to help remove them from the body), and his symptoms virtually cleared up within three months. Fortunately, Matthew's parents were hesitant to start him on Ritalin for the ADD, which, in retrospect, probably would have been of no help anyhow, since it was lead poisoning that was causing his problem.

Lead Paint Testing and Removal: Leave It to a Professional

If you suspect your home may be contaminated with lead, testing and, if necessary, removal (called abatement) should be done only by a professional. Home testing kits to check for lead in paint, soil, and dust are not recommended by federal agencies at this time.[11]

There are two basic methods of looking for lead in paint. The first method is X-ray fluorescence, which involves the use of a portable detector that X-rays a painted surface and measures the amount of lead in all the layers of the paint. Since different paint may have been used in different rooms, all painted surfaces should be checked. The second method is the laboratory testing of paint samples, which involves the removal of about two inches of the suspect paint for testing. To test for lead dust in the soil around your home, samples should be taken and sent to a laboratory.

Remember, lead is a known neurotoxin. It can damage the brains of young children at levels that have not been clearly defined. It can also damage the kidneys and affect the blood pressure and the immune and cardiovascular systems of both children and adults.[12] Prenatal exposures can cause lower birth weight, spontaneous abortion, and poor mental development. Whatever effort you take to make sure your children's environment is as lead-free as possible will help assure that their future is as bright as possible—and is one of the best gifts you can give them.

CAN YOU THINK AND PAINT AT THE SAME TIME?

Toxic metals such as lead and mercury are no longer allowed in paint. However, reading the labels on the cans of some types of paint will still reveal warnings about other toxic substances, such as solvents, which can cause brain damage.

The Franklin Institute asks, in an article on the history of lead, why painting has long been such a toxic activity. "For some reason, paint seems to be the delivery system of choice for brain damage. Will future archeologists be baffled by a society whose walls were more vibrant than its brain cells?"

MERCURY: THE NEUROTOXIC NIGHTMARE THAT HAUNTS OUR DAILY LIVES

While it is now believed that the brain-destroying "mad cow disease" can be spread to humans through infected beef, precisely how it works is still largely a mystery. But there's no mystery as to the cause of the "mad fish disease" that ravaged the brains of thousands of people living in postwar Japan. It was mercury, the highly neurotoxic heavy metal, which became bioconcentrated in the seafood that was Japan's principal source of protein as a result of industrial pollution.

The mass mercury poisoning that affected the inhabitants of the town of Minamata and environs during the mid-1950s was a first of sorts. Up to then, mercury poisoning had mainly been the result of occupational exposures (from which the term "mad as a hatter" originated). But in Minamata, all the conditions for such a catastrophic event came together. The town's dominant industry, a petrochemical plant owned by the Chisso Corporation, had been dumping toxic waste into the adjacent bay for years and had been opting to pay off the local fishermen whose livelihoods were being impacted rather than find a safer method of disposal. Among the hazardous wastes were the mercury compounds used in the manufacture of a chemical called acetaldehyde. And as its sales steadily increased, even through the war, the plant, as well as the surrounding population from which it recruited its workers, grew.

But in 1956, a doctor working for the company hospital reported that "an unclarified disease of the central nervous system has broken out." In fact, scores of people had begun developing devastating symptoms, ranging from slurred speech and tunnel vision to splitting headaches, numbness of the limbs and lips, uncontrollable shouting, involuntary movements, and loss of consciousness. Moreover, cats in the town were thought to have gone crazy, and birds began dropping from the sky. Eventually, more than 900 people died of what became known as "Minamata disease." But because of a company cover-up and small payoffs to victims, the poisoning of Minamata Bay and those who lived near it continued for another twelve years. And only recently, a study by doctors at Kumamoto University revealed that tens of thousands more people may have been affected by this brain shattering "disease" than was previously believed. If ever anyone wanted proof of the power of mercury not only to kill, but to utterly destroy the quality of people's lives, they need look no further than the Minamata disaster.

Mercury is a pernicious poison that can wreak havoc on the brain and central nervous system, as well as on the liver and kidneys. Furthermore, it accumulates in the environment. Because of this, the U.S. Agency for Toxic Substances and Disease registry lists mercury as third on its most hazardous substances list.

But that hasn't stopped us from making this incredibly dangerous and tricky substance an intrinsic part of our daily lives, with the sources of exposure ranging from dental fillings and fever thermometers to batteries and fluorescent lights to power plant emissions. We even routinely inject it into our newborns and toddlers, a practice that, as we shall see, has now been linked to a sharp rise in brain disorders.

That's why, in your efforts to protect your family from the effects of toxic chemicals, mercury is one that you simply can't afford to ignore.

Do Your Kids Really Need a Mouthful of Mercury?

If you or your kids have ever had a cavity, it's quite likely that you or they have one or more silver (amalgam) fillings—perhaps even a whole bunch. It may therefore come as a surprise to learn that the safety of amalgams (a term that actually means "mixed with mercury") has been suspect since the introduction of the mixture as a filling material more than 150 years ago. Concerns about its safety have by no means been resolved since then.

The concept that mercury leaks from silver fillings—especially during the consumption of hot foods and beverages, and while chewing gum—and may be the catalyst in a wide variety of health problems is not a new one. Originally, the American Society of Dental Surgeons, predecessor of the American Dental Association (ADA), actually had its members pledge not to use amalgam. But the ADA, founded in 1859, took the opposite position, and has continued to regard any suggestion that amalgam may be hazardous as professional heresy.

Despite that, a growing number of health experts are beginning to question the wisdom of having a mouthful of toxic metal. Several years ago, in fact, Canadian health officials issued a position statement recommending that dentists in Canada use non-mercury fillings for children, pregnant women, and people with impaired kidney function.

Considering what we already know about the dangers of mercury poisoning, those sound like good suggestions for non-Canadians as well. But you have to make a point of telling your child's (and your own) dentist that you don't want amalgams, and not let him or her convince you that they're really harmless. Just remember: Keeping mercury out of your children's teeth (and your own) in the first place is a whole lot easier than later having it removed.

Should you decide to have the amalgams in your mouth extracted, however, remember that it's extremely important to have the work done by a highly competent and experienced professional in this particular area, or you could well end up ingesting a lot of that mercury you're trying to get rid of. And if you're pregnant, forget about it until after the baby arrives.

Got Mercury?

Even though mercury thermometers are probably not for sale in your drugstore anymore, you might still have one in your bathroom medicine cabinet. Mercury thermometers are made of glass and contain a silvery white liquid, which is the mercury. An average thermometer contains about 1 gram of mercury, which is enough to contaminate a 20-acre lake and thereby require fish advisories, according to Michael Bender, director of the Mercury Policy Project, which was formed to raise awareness of mercury contamination. If you still have a mercury thermometer, you should replace it immediately with a digital, glass alcohol, or infrared ear thermometer. Do not throw your mercury thermometer in the trash, however! Find out where your town collects hazardous waste and drop it off.

If your mercury thermometer breaks, you will need to clean up the mercury promptly and correctly. If you don't clean up the spill, it will evaporate, possibly contaminating the indoor air with dangerous levels of mercury. The smaller and more poorly ventilated the room is, the higher the risk that dangerous levels will be reached.[13]

If your thermometer breaks:

- Keep people and pets out of the area.
- Try to keep the area as cool as possible. Turn off any heaters and turn up the air conditioner.
- Get as much ventilation in the room as possible. If you can, keep the windows open for at least two days.
- Do not use a vacuum or broom to clean up the spill.
- Do not touch the mercury! Remove all the jewelry and watches from your hands, as the mercury will bond with the metal, and wear rubber gloves.
- Use a flashlight to locate the mercury. The light will reflect off the beads and make them easier to find.
- On a hard surface, use stiff paper to push the beads together. Use an eyedropper to suction the beads of mercury up, or working over a tray to catch any spills, lift the beads up with the stiff paper. Carefully place the beads in a wide-mouth container, then pick up any remaining beads with wide duct or packaging tape. Put the contaminated tape, eyedropper, paper, and gloves in a plastic bag and seal. Place the plastic bag, along with the wide-mouth container, in a second bag and seal. Label the bag as "mercury waste," and call your state agency for disposal information.
- On a carpet or rug, cut out the contaminated section and seal it in a plastic bag labeled as "mercury waste." Call your state agency for disposal information.
- In a sink of water, the mercury will sink to the bottom, so you must remove as much of the water as possible and then recover the mercury with an eyedropper. Put the mercury in a wide-mouth container, close the lid, and seal the container

with strong tape. Label the container as "mercury waste," and call your state agency for disposal instructions.

- If the mercury goes down the drain, it will get caught in your sink trap. You must remove the trap and, working over a tray, pour its contents into a wide-mouth container. Close the container with the lid and seal it with strong tape. Label the container as "mercury waste," and call your state agency for disposal instructions.
- If you are pregnant, have someone else do the cleanup.

Testing the Metal of an "Autistic" Child

Michael was two years old when his mother first brought him to see Dr. Magaziner and when he had already been labeled with possible autism or pervasive developmental delay (PDD). Michael had progressed normally to eighteen months, but somewhere between eighteen and twenty-four months, he lost the desire to make eye contact, became withdrawn, and started toe walking. He also stopped using the words he had previously learned, and his speech development came to a halt.

Michael's parents were worried that mercury in his immunizations may have triggered these problems (see "Vaccinations: An Ounce of Prevention or a Ton of Trouble?" on page 200). A month prior to seeing Dr. Magaziner, they started him on a dairy-free diet, since they had read that dairy products are often improperly processed in autistic children, and began giving him a multivitamin-and-mineral supplement, as well as B_{12}, folic acid, and cod liver oil supplements.

Testing of urine and stool samples by Dr. Magaziner revealed not only high levels of mercury in the child's body, but of tin and nickel as well. All three are neurotoxic and can affect brain function. Possible sources of nickel exposure for toddlers include cigarette smoke, chocolate, and hydrogenated oils. Tin can be found in drinking water and some toothpaste, as well as in dyes and bleaching agents. Many toxic metals are also present in our environment due to pollution. They are found in the air we breathe,

the water we drink, and the food we eat. At two, Michael's detoxification pathways were not mature yet, so his body could not excrete these poisons.

Because Michael had been on numerous courses of antibiotics, he was also found to have an overgrowth of yeast in his intestinal tract. Dr. Magaziner frequently diagnoses and treats children with yeast infections and dysbiosis.

Michael's treatments consisted of a chelating agent to remove the mercury, tin, and nickel; an antifungal for the yeast overgrowth; supplemental glutathione, an enzyme that stimulates the liver detoxification pathways and attacks free radicals; and probiotics, coenzyme Q10 (CoQ10), and extra vitamin C. He was also taken off foods containing gluten, a protein found in wheat, barley, and oats. A lot of kids, particularly ones who have taken frequent courses of antibiotics, cannot effectively break down certain food proteins in their stomachs and benefit from the removal of casein and gluten from their diets. These proteins, known as polypeptides, can form in the gastrointestinal tract, circulate to the brain, and trigger abnormal forms of behavior.

Michael's levels of mercury, tin, and nickel steadily declined after he was put on this course of treatment; he became much more aware of his surroundings, was able to be potty trained, and in six months, went from saying no words to speaking full sentences. In fact, his mother calls him "almost a normal child now."

Unfortunately, Michael's case is not all that unique. Dr. Magaziner has seen and treated many similar cases. But the good news is that such children can show great improvement once their imbalances have been corrected.

All too often, a child is labeled as having a certain condition or infirmity; he or she will be called autistic, for example, and that's the way he or she will come to be regarded. The real question, however, should be: What's causing the condition? What factors might possibly be triggering the problem, and is there something that can be done to eliminate them? Perhaps rather than simply being dismissed as one more possible case of autism, Michael should have been diagnosed with metal toxicity.

It should be incumbent on a physician, when faced with a case such as Michael's, to start doing some investigative work and look at other possibilities, such as the child's environment, diet, vaccination history, and previous medical treatments. But all too often, doctors are not trained to thoroughly evaluate each child's unique biochemistry, and instead, hasten to give the condition a convenient label (for example, autistic spectrum disorder). That's why it's more essential than ever for parents to be aware of environmental and dietary triggers for health problems and to seek out practitioners who have interest, training, and experience in environmental and nutritional medicine.

Fortunately, there are a few hundred doctors who, like Dr. Magaziner, have been trained to use the Defeat Autism Now! (DAN!) protocol in evaluating and treating children who have been labeled with PDD or an autistic spectrum disorder. To find a doctor in your area, contact the Autism Research Institute or the American College for Advancement in Medicine (see "Resources" at the end of this chapter).

Vaccinations: An Ounce of Prevention or a Ton of Trouble?

Once upon a time, not so very long ago, medical professionals were pretty much assumed to know what they were talking about. If a doctor made a diagnosis or said something was needed, that was good enough for the vast majority of people. And one of the things that was needed, according to doctors, was for children to be immunized against specific diseases, most notably smallpox and, later on, polio, a scourge that killed or crippled numerous children during the first half of the twentieth century.

But while both those serious diseases have virtually disappeared in recent years, vaccinations have not, and more and more of them have been developed against all manner of common childhood illnesses and are almost always required as a condition of entry to public school. Some of these have been combined into "supershots," administered in a single visit to the doctor's office. Most family physicians and pediatricians continue to claim that this is all well and good, as do professional groups such as the American Medical Association (AMA). But increasingly, people are no longer willing to take their word for it, particularly a growing number of parents who have witnessed terrible changes in their children's health and personalities that they say occurred following these multivaccination sessions.

Supporting these parents in that conviction are the results of recent research, which indicate that there may well be links between the way vaccines are formulated and administered and the notable rise in cases of childhood autism and related conditions, including ADD. (According to FDA statistics, the cases of autism in the United States have nearly reached the 500,000 mark, or almost 1 in every 250 infants, representing an increase of more than 500 percent in the last decade.)

One such vaccine ingredient is mercury, which is known to cause neurological, immunological, sensory, motor, and behavioral disabilities, problems often identical to the symptoms observed in "autistic" children. Mercury is among the components of thimerosal, a preservative long used in a considerable number of vaccines, including diphtheria-pertussis-tetanus (DPT) and hepatitis B shots. Despite official claims that the amount of mercury involved poses no significant hazard, the concerns raised did prompt the FDA to strongly recommend the removal of thimerosal from new batches of vaccine. However, the old ones have not been recalled and remain in use.

Had the controversy not literally "hit home" for a prominent legislator, however, the agency might not have felt pressured to take even that action. "I don't have to read a letter to experience the heartbreak. I see it in my own family," noted Indiana Congressman Dan Burton in opening remarks to a hearing of the Government Reform Committee on Autism, which he chaired in April 2000. Burton went on to relate how his grandson Christian, whom he described as having been a healthy and beautiful child who was "outgoing and talkative," had gone into an autistic state virtually overnight following a visit to the doctor's office during which he was given a number of routine immunizations.

That night Christian had a slight fever and he slept for long periods of time. When he was awake he would scream a horrible high-pitched scream. He would scream for hours. He began dragging his head on the furniture and banging it repeatedly. Over the week-and-a-half after the vaccinations, Christian would stare into space and act like he was deaf. He would hit himself and others, which was something he had never done. He would shake his head from side to side as fast as he could. He lost all language.

In recounting his own family's ordeal, Burton emphasized that he was not against vaccinations and didn't think they were responsible for all cases of autism. "However," he added, "there is enough evidence emerging of some kind of a connection for some children that we can't close our eyes to it. We have to learn more."[14]

Nor is mercury seen as the only possible culprit in this connection. Another combined-vaccine formula known as the MMR—for measles, mumps, and rubella—is also believed by many to be a suspect in cases of autism, particularly following a study of a small group of autistic children led by Andrew Wakefield, M.D., a gastroenterologist from London's Royal Free Hospital and School of Medicine, and published in the British medical journal *The Lancet*. All of the children had intestinal problems that Wakefield's research suggested were associated with the vaccine, based on a finding of measles virus in the gut wall that it was hypothesized could have also had an adverse effect on brain function.

The latter findings stirred a heated debate, particularly after they were publicized on the CBS newsmagazine *60 Minutes*, with the AMA and other defenders of conventional medical wisdom making a point of attempting to discredit Wakefield's research and to reassure the public that the MMR vaccine is no cause for concern. "To date, there have been no convincing scientific data that links any vaccine to autism or any other kind of behavioral disorder," contended the AMA in a press release, which included the DPT vaccine in the assessment. Furthermore, it noted, "A working group convened by the National Institutes of Health concluded in 1995 that autism is a genetic condition," and a more recent article in *Scientific American* concluded that the condition may be due to "malfunctioning genes" producing "subtle changes in the structure of the brain stem." More recently, a Danish study comparing children who had received the vaccine with those who hadn't concluded that the risk of autism was similar for both groups. "The AMA believes that critical public health decisions must be made on the basis of well-conducted scientific research and established scientific fact, and not on anecdotal case reports," the group's release declared.

But to many parents, the anecdotal experience of seeing seemingly healthy, well-adjusted children suddenly descend into a twilight world of bizarre behavior after being given multiple inoculations is evidence enough that "autism" isn't necessarily a genetic condition, but may be directly related to what's in those vaccines. Also convinced of that are a number of lawyers who have agreed to represent them, at least in regard to the mercury issue. In April 2002, a class action lawsuit against the manufacturers of thimerosal and the vaccine manufacturers who used it was filed in the U.S. District Court for the Eastern District of New York based on claims that the amounts of mercury contained in these vaccines far exceeded the levels considered "safe" by the EPA.

The safety of these MMR vaccinations has also continued to be called into question. "Thousands of parents believe that the MMR vaccine has contributed to their children's autism," noted longtime pediatrician and vaccine researcher F. Edward Yazbak, M.D., of Falmouth, Massachusetts. "They speak of the MMR being the only new event in their child's life in that period between normal development and autistic regression . . . These parents certainly did not acquire their conviction from reading about the twelve cases reported in Dr. Wakefield's first paper . . .

[A]lways remember their children were normal and their disease is acquired."

Noting that such parents no longer believe health authorities' assurances that the vaccine is safe, Dr. Yazbak also charged that "the infectious disease specialists and epidemiologists who make decisions and mandate vaccines have little knowledge of autism and its immune etiology."

Another critic, Dr. Tedd Koren, a Pennsylvania-based chiropractor and author of *Childhood Vaccination: Questions All Parents Should Ask* (Koren Publications, 2000), charges that doctors routinely fail to report vaccine reactions because "they don't want to, they don't recognize it, and they're afraid of malpractice. The truth is, we don't know how many kids are being hurt."

Koren even disputes the conventional medicine position that vaccinations are necessary to protect against childhood diseases (or as one pediatric Web site puts it, that "without immunizations, your child can catch diseases that may cause high fever, coughing, choking, breathing problems and even brain injury" that "may leave your child deaf or blind, cause paralysis and even death.") "If we stopped vaccinating, we would not have an outbreak of measles tomorrow," says Dr. Koren. Rather, "we would stop having an outbreak or epidemic of autism," which Dr. Koren claims has corresponded with the increased use of vaccines. "You didn't see autism in Japan until after World War II, when the Americans instituted an immunization program," he says.

"When you eat fish, it's ingested; when you get a vaccine with mercury, it's injected," observes Koren, adding, "Stop with the tuna already."

All of which could pose a real dilemma for you as a parent concerned about protecting your kids. Should you put your faith in the assurances of conventional medicine and health authorities, or be genuinely alarmed by the anecdotal reports of children becoming autistic following inoculations? And if the latter, should you carry it to the point of challenging the immunization policy of your local school district, if necessary?

That's a question only you can answer and a decision in which your parenting instinct and your "sixth sense" will have to be your guides. But while contemplating the pros and cons of this issue, there are a few points you might want to keep in mind:

- Whatever you decide to do, do it because you truly believe it's in the best interest of your child, not simply to "cooperate with" or please those in authority.

- Multiple shots are administered for cost-efficiency, not health reasons (despite the various rationales used for giving them, such as the argument that the child might not be brought back for subsequent shots). If you're concerned about the effects of all those different vaccines being given to your child in one visit, tell the doctor that you want them spread out.

- You might want to evaluate the need for each immunization individually, decide whether you think it's really warranted, and convey that decision to your doctor or hospital. What are the chances, for instance, that your child will contract hepatitis B, a disease associated with sexual transmission and needles used in injecting illicit drugs?

- Then, too, rather than having your child vaccinated during infancy, you might want to wait until his or her immune system has developed to some degree.

- Perhaps most important, you can insist that any vaccine used on your child be from a new batch that doesn't contain mercury in the form of thimerosal. Any way you cut it, mercury is a highly toxic substance and, whether or not the amounts used in vaccines cause autism, is not the sort of thing that goes with raising chemical-free kids.

Heavy metals are apt to be damaging in their effects, but there are definite steps you can take to keep your children from being exposed to them. The effort is not one that you should put off, particularly if you have any reason at all to suspect that your kids' environment may be harboring a source of such exposure. Time is of essence, and the sooner you eliminate any such hazard, the less chance it will put your children's future at risk.

Resources

Lead

Alliance to End Childhood Lead Poisoning
Web site: www.aeclp.org
News, solutions, legal remedies, and resources to help parents with lead issues.

Citizens' Lead Education and Poisoning Prevention
Web site: www.clepp.org
The Web site of the nonprofit community organization of Birmingham, Alabama, dedicated to community education, hazard control training, and policy changes.

National Lead Information Center
Web site: www.epa.gov/lead/nlic.htm
Information for the general public and professionals about lead hazards and their prevention.

The Maine Lead Action Project
Web site: www.maineleadaction.org
The Web site of the Maine Lead Action Project, which is working for the elimination of childhood lead poisoning through education, support, assistance, and encouragement to families and communities in Maine.

Mercury

Autism and Mercury
Web site: www.autism-mercury.com

Discussion, articles, letters, and links related to the possible cause-and-effect relationship between mercury and autism.

Mercury Policy Project
Web site: www.mercurypolicy.org
A Web site promoting policies to eliminate mercury uses, reduce its export, and significantly reduce mercury exposures at local, national, and international levels.

Physician Referrals

American College for Advancement in Medicine (ACAM)
23121 Verdugo Drive
Suite 204
Laguna Hills, CA 92653
Telephone: 800-532-3688
Web site: www.acam.org
Referrals to nutritionally oriented physicians.

Vaccinations and Autism

Autism Research Institute and Defeat Autism Now! (DAN!)
Web site: www.autism.com/ari/contents.html
The Web site of the nonprofit organization devoted to conducting and disseminating research on the causes of autism and on methods of preventing, diagnosing, and treating autism and other severe behavioral disorders of childhood.

Koren Publications, Inc.
Web site: www.korenpublications.com
Sells Dr. Tedd Koren's book *Childhood Vaccinations: Questions All Parents Should Ask.*

PART THREE

FOOD FIT FOR A KID

❅ **7** ❅

Organically Grown Solutions

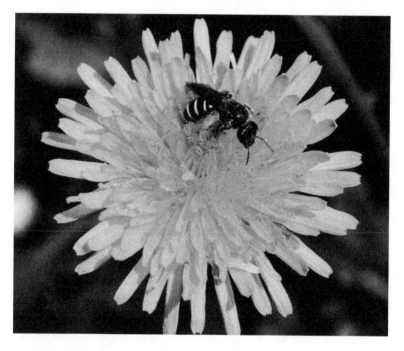

"I went over to a huge farm that produces hundreds of bushels of tomatoes . . . beautiful plants, not a weed in them . . . all of a sudden I thought: What's wrong here? There was not a bird or a bee or a fly . . . but there were these huge trucks with giant tanks spraying the pesticides and the herbicides."
—Marge Ratliff, organic farmer

WHAT YOU'LL FIND IN THIS CHAPTER

Where have the vitamins and minerals gone? Fresh vegetables may look the same as they did in the 1970s, but as far as their nutrient content goes, things have changed. It seems that certain vegetables grown at the end of the 1990s had significantly less amounts of iron, calcium, vitamin A, and Vitamin C than those grown twenty-two years ago. Why were these nutrients missing? The USDA says it doesn't know. However, experts have suggested that chemically based agriculture robs soil of its fertility, and that poor soil, in turn, produces inferior crops.

SOS: Save Our Soil. If you think of soil not just as dirt, but rather as a living, fertile medium for producing a nutritious and delicious bounty without dependence on harmful chemicals, you won't think much of conventional agriculture. Organic farming, by contrast, is based on the concept of healthy soil that's been "detoxified." Soil does have the ability to overcome chemical addiction and actually gets better each year that it's organically farmed.

Organically grown food offers numerous benefits. Not only are organic products grown without toxic chemicals and fertilizers, but the land in which they're grown must be free of prohibited substances for a minimum of three years. Detailed records must be kept that can track the finished products all the way back to the farm. Organic convenience foods, such as granola bars, cookies, and corn chips, do not contain the chemical additives that are common in conventional food, such as aspartame, hydrogenated oils, and artificial preservatives and colors. The implementation of the national organic standards, which went into effect in October 2002, means that all labeled organic products, not just products "certified organic," must be produced according to the same standards. And when you see the organic label on packaged and convience foods, it's your assurance that they've been manufactured without such unhealthy additives as hydrogenated oils, petroleum-based artificial colors, and synthetic preservatives. It's the one way you can allow your kids to have convenience foods, yet still keep their diet free of chemicals.

Things You Can Do Now!

- Support organic farming by asking your retailer to stock organic products. Vote for safe, nutritious food and good agricultural practices by how you spend your dollars.
- Not only can you eat organically grown food, but you can wear organic clothing as well. Support the earth with the shirt on your back.
- Think locally. Start by setting an example in your own front yard and stop using chemical pesticides and fertilizers. Cancel the visits from the lawn "care" companies. Dandelions are beneficial plants, not public enemy number one.
- Even if you don't have a lot of space, you can start your own "organic garden" with at least one container of organic tomatoes or a window box of organic herbs.

The invisible differences between conventionally and organically grown commodities and ingredients may not seem to matter all that much. But as it turns out, those differences go far deeper than most parents may ever have realized. In addition to exposing kids and adults to a variety of poisons that tend to accumulate and interact in the body, chemically cultivated foods may well deprive our children of the nutrients so essential to good health (and have adverse effects on the environment as well). Another advantage in choosing organic foods is that they don't contain any artificial colorings, flavorings, preservatives, artificial sweeteners, or partially hydrogenated oils. You might even be able to leave your label-reading glasses at home! What it all boils down to is a choice between foods that are quite possibly less beneficial than they used to be and in all probability contain traces of toxic chemicals, and essentially poison-free foods that are apt to have retained a higher nutritional value.

Once you understand these differences, the choices you make will all fall into place. Of course, in an age dominated by convenience foods and busy schedules, implementing them may require some planning and organization. The suggestions and guidelines in this chapter are designed to assist you in directing your family's eating habits toward that goal.

THE CASE OF THE MISSING NUTRIENTS

It was a case of "mysterious disappearance" that had profound implications for the American public (and especially kids). During the twenty-two years between 1975 and 1997, at least a dozen types of fresh vegetables grown in the United States had lost a substantial amount of their vitamin and mineral content.

This dietary whodunit might never have come to light had it not been for an analysis of USDA nutrient data performed by the Kushi Institute of Becket, Massachusetts. What it found was that the nutritional value of the vegetables being grown at the close of the twentieth century was significantly less than that of vegetables available a quarter century earlier. According to the calculations, the average calcium level in the twelve veggies analyzed was down 27 percent; the average iron level, 37 percent; the average vitamin A level, 21 percent; and the average vitamin C level, 30 percent.

Now, one might think that the disclosure of so vast a vanishing act would send federal investigators scurrying into action. But when contacted by *Organic Gardening* magazine, USDA scientist David Haytowitz is reported to have said that he did "not know the cause . . . and that his office does not have responsibility to investigate this issue." Haytowitz was not aware of anyone else at the agency who might have an answer to the enigma.[1]

As it turned out, however, it wasn't just the United States that was victimized by the vegetable devaluation. The case of the missing nutrients soon became one of international intrigue as well. That same year, a report in the *British Food Journal* noted that in the fifty years between 1930 and 1980, some twenty food crops analyzed had suffered similar losses, including a 19 percent decline in calcium, a 22 percent loss of iron, and a 14 percent drop in potassium levels.[2] Only, the author of this particular report, Anne-Marie Mayer (now at Cornell University), had a theory to offer—that the disappearance was quite likely linked to changes in agricultural practices, including soil compaction, the use of agricultural chemicals, disruption of soil life, and deficiencies in organic matter.

The editors of *Organic Gardening* magazine go even further in posing a solution to this mystery. They strongly suspect the culprit to be chemically based agriculture, which they believe has succeeded in robbing crops of nutrients by depleting the soil in which they're grown of its fertility. Stop using chemicals, they suggest.

In proposing this solution, the *Organic Gardening* editors cite other corroborative evidence: A 1999 report on an ongoing thirty-seven-year project at the University of Wisconsin–Madison concluded that overapplication of nitrogen fertilizers is irreparably damaging the fertility of soil, causing it in effect to age the equivalent of 5,000 years. (This excess nitrogen, they also point out, is a major perpetrator in the pollution of lakes, streams, and groundwater.)[3]

For mothers who have attempted every type of scheme and strategy to get kids to eat their vegetables, such reports that today's produce may have been looted of much of its benefits are apt to be discouraging indeed. The good news, however, is that not all veggies are victims of such nutritional fleecing. There are some that have been endowed with a kind of built-in security system to help them keep their vitamin and mineral assets intact—those that are organically grown.

SAVING OUR SOIL FROM CHEMICAL ADDICTION

For most consumers, the term "organic" used to describe food has come to mean that it was grown without any toxic pesticides or chemical fertilizers. That's true, but it doesn't define the broader meaning of the word, which offers a more complete understanding of its application to crop cultivation. In its more complete sense, "organic" refers to a system of sustainable agriculture that is very much the opposite of the fragmented, short-sighted farming techniques that have reduced both the safety and the quality of our conventional food supply.

The use of the word "organic" in this regard goes back at least sixty years, when it was first believed to have been used in the book *Look to the Land*, written by Lord Northbourn. In this book, Lord Northbourn envisioned the farm as "a dynamic, living, balanced organic whole, or an organism." This principle is similar to the one behind the science of ecology—the study of the relationships between organisms—and in fact, is now the basis of a related field that applies the concept to farming, called agroecology.[4]

At the heart of the organic orientation is a reverence for the soil itself, the idea that the soil must be handled with care to continue producing a nutrition-rich bounty, rather than being abused, exploited, and worn out, as it now is by the "agribusiness" culture that has largely replaced the old-fashioned family farm. It's why the goals of the Rodale Institute of Kutztown, Pennsylvania, which has been a leading force in promoting and researching regenerative agriculture, include increasing public awareness "that healthy food can only be obtained from healthy soil" and making soil quality "as important to the public as air and water quality."[5]

In essence, the primary mission of organic farming is to save the soil that produces the food on which we depend for our very survival. Those who profit from the use of agricultural chemicals like to claim that they're the ones responsible for our food supply's preservation and abundance. This was asserted several years ago on the network newsmagazine show *20/20* by celebrity correspondent John Stossel. His premise that organic produce is no safer than conventional varieties, and may even be more hazardous, was later shown to be based on fraudulent test results, leading to an on-air apology by Stossel.

What's actually happening is the creation of chemically addicted soil that is slowly but surely poisoning the planet from the ground up. Oft-repeated assertions that organic growing methods are "not a viable option" because they can't compete with conventional, chemical-based agriculture in terms of yield simply don't jibe with the actual results achieved by organic farmers and experimental facilities like the Rodale Institute. In 1989, for instance, the National Research Council reported that the average yields of eight organic farms it studied were generally equal to or better than those of the surrounding conventional farms—without the cost (both monetary and environmental) of synthetic chemicals. In addition, organic crops have been found to be far more resilient in their ability to withstand the effects of drought and bad weather conditions.[6]

What the organic farmer strives to do is to eliminate the bad habits that have proven so injurious to the land and its occupants and to restore the healthy ones engaged in by our forefathers (as well as to introduce some newer, more sophisticated interpretations of our forefathers' ideas). One of the techniques used to achieve this is crop rotation. According to the Rodale Institute's farm manager, Jeff Moyer, the lack of diversity in crop cultivation seen on conventional farms is "not healthy and can't be sustained naturally. In organic agriculture, by contrast, we're not just trying to grow a crop, we're trying to grow soil." And soil, much like people, can be "rehabilitated," Moyer says. It eventually regenerates itself if allowed to grow a variety of crops and if kept free of chemicals. The idea behind soil rehabilitation is that "the soil wants to be covered with something green and growing all the time," says Moyer. "If you have a little garden patch and you do nothing with it, it's going to get covered with weeds."[7]

Other organic procedures include the release of beneficial insects that prey on pests, eliminating the need for toxic and polluting insecticides, and the use of composted manure (processed for safety in accord with strict rules) and vegetable matter to fertilize the soil naturally. At the root of such practices is the concept that healthy soil grows healthier plants, and healthier plants are more resistant to pest infestation.

While it may seem a no-brainer that organic foods have fewer pesticide residues than their conventionally grown counterparts, up until a report released in May 2002, it appears no one had officially compared the two. The study, done by teams from both the Consumers Union (CU) and the Organic Materials Research Institute (OMRI), found that 73 percent of the conventionally grown foods tested had at least one pesticide residue, while only 23 percent of the organically grown samples (of the same crop) had any such residues. The research disclosed that 90 percent of the USDA samples of conventionally grown apples, peaches, pears, strawberries, and celery had residues, with the nonorganic crops being one-sixth as likely to contain multiple pesticide residues.[8]

But why do organic crops contain any pesticide residue at all? Some of the residues picked up in the testing were the result of banned, but very persistent, chemicals: organochlorine insecticides, including DDT, which are still in the soil despite the fact they are no longer allowed to be used in the United States. When those chemicals were excluded from the data, the organic crops with residues dropped from 23 percent to 13 percent. The remaining residues were explained by past soil contamination, pesticide drift, and possibly mislabeled conventional crops posing as organic. One of the report's coauthors, Edward Groth III, senior scientist at the CU, said the study shows that consumers who buy organic food are exposed to "one-third as many residues as they'd eat in conventionally grown food, and the residues are usually lower as well."

Previous studies by the CU found that certain nonorganic foods, such as apples, peaches, spinach, and green beans, had residues of numerous pesticides (at relatively high levels), while other conventionally grown crops, including, bananas, broccoli, carrots, and fruit juices, had fewer and lower residues.

If you've been serving your family organic foods without waiting for such a study to prove what common sense should tell you is true, you're one up on the scientists.

A Pesticide By Any Other Name . . .

-cide/-side/suffix. 1. Killer. Derived from Latin, "to kill."
All chemical "-cides" are legally considered pesticides. However,
each has its killing specialty:

Insecticides—pesticides that kill insects.
Herbicides—pesticides that kill plants.
Fungicides—pesticides that kill molds.
Rodenticides—pesticides that kill rodents.

What the "Organic" Label Promises

Earning organic certification for a commodity requires a producer to adhere to some rigorous standards, starting with a three-year wait for the field in which the food is grown to be certified organic. (Three years is the time required for a field to be "detoxed" of any previous chemical use.) The process also calls for meticulous and complete record-keeping. "It all starts on the farm," is how a representative of the Organic Trade Association, based in Greenfield, Massachusetts, explains it. "Everything else that happens along the chain of production is done to preserve the organic integrity that started on the farm."

These criteria are all spelled out under the new federal labeling regulation, one that might have allowed the definition of "organic" to be corrupted had it not been for the efforts of many dedicated people to ensure that earlier versions that would have weakened the concept were rejected. While the final rule exempts farms and organizations selling less than $5,000 in organic produce per year from having to be certified, it does require them to comply with the same standards or face possible penalties. That's not to say, however, that such standards didn't previously exist—in fact, more than thirty state and private agencies offered organic certification prior to adoption of the new regulation, which was authorized by passage of the Organic Foods Production Act of 1990.

Organic certification means:

- A prohibition on the use of toxic and persistent chemicals in the soil for at least three years prior to the harvesting of an organic crop (which doesn't ensure that a commodity will be entirely pesticide-free, as the CU study showed, since it may come into contact with pesticides carried on the wind or residues of long-term chemicals remaining in soil).
- A ban on the use of sewage sludge as fertilizer, the genetic engineering of crops, and irradiation to kill pathogens (all of which would have been allowed under the original proposed regulation).
- Preferred use of organic seed and plant stock, with non-organic varieties permitted under certain conditions.
- Use of various physical, mechanical, and biological forms of pest control, with certain synthetic substances from a specific approved list allowed if those methods prove insufficient.
- A ban on antibiotic and synthetic hormone use in cattle, along with a requirement that the cattle be fed 100 percent organic feed (with some vitamins permitted) and given access to pasture.
- A requirement that convenience foods labeled "100 percent organic" must be just that; that foods labeled "organic" must contain at least 95 percent organic ingredients; and that products that are 70 to 95 percent organic must be labeled "made with organic ingredients."
- A requirement that the chemical additives commonly used in conventional food, such as aspartame, hydrogenated oils, artificial preservatives, and coloring agents, are not used.
- A requirement that all those who process and handle organic products are certified by a USDA-accredited certification agency.
- A mandatory certification and inspection of both the farms

where raw commodities or ingredients are grown and the facilities that produce processed organic foods.

- Detailed record-keeping on the materials and processes used in all phases of organic food production, with documentation assuring that the organic products are not comingled with nonorganic ones.

As you can see, this new legislation strives to provide consumers with a clear definition of the term "organic."

INERT? NOT EXACTLY

Have you ever looked at the label of a pesticide product? You'll find two basic ingredient types: active and inert. The active ingredients are those developed to kill (or harm) a pest. All the other ingredients added to facilitate the product's usage are inert.

While the label of "inert" implies chemical inactivity, often these ingredients are anything but. According to the Northwest Coalition for Alternatives to Pesticides (NCAP), which has researched inert ingredients, the evidence shows that many are hazardous to our health and the environment. The trouble is, the identities of such ingredients are often claimed to be confidential by the pesticide manufacturers and not disclosed on the label.

According to NCAP, more than a quarter of inert ingredients (or about 600 chemicals) are classified as hazardous by state, federal, and international agencies.[9] So there's more to a pesticide label than meets the eye.

CREATING YOUR OWN ORGANIC GARDEN

"More in a garden grows than what the gardener sows," goes a Spanish proverb. A garden can delight the eye from a distance with blooms and numerous shades of green, and from up close with the gentle radiance contained in a single drop of water perched on a leaf. A garden can be your place of retreat or just some pots brightening up a patio. Whatever a garden is, or can be, to you and your kids, it should definitely not be a place to spray toxic chemicals. Your garden should be a welcome spot for bees and birds; a place to observe a spider's web spun across two branches or a small toad hiding in the soil. Keep your garden a place for nature to unfold naturally, without chemical odors or areas unsafe for kids, and whatever you grow will be as much a delight to the earth as it is to you.

Where to Start

First think "sunny soil." You'll want to pick a location for your vegetable garden that receives at least six to eight hours of sunlight a day. It should also have well-drained soil. By that we mean an area that doesn't form puddles after a rainstorm. To determine whether your proposed spot has sufficient drainage, examine it immediately after a rainstorm. Choose your location well, and you'll avoid problems after you've gone to the trouble of planting.

The other important thing you can do before planting is to have the soil from the location you've selected tested for nutrient levels. (If you're concerned about possible environmental contamination of the soil, you can also have it tested for a variety of toxins. However, testing for toxins is much more costly than testing for nutrients.) Nutrient testing is inexpensive and can be done by most agricultural extension offices for approximately $8 to $25. Some garden shops sell nutrient-testing kits as well. Such testing enables you to know what "ingredients" your soil needs to be properly enriched.

Richard VanVranken, agricultural agent for the Rutgers Cooperative Extension Service in Atlantic County, New Jersey, often hears from people who "just throw seeds in the ground without doing anything to the soil." Their plants come up "sickly and yellow and they think the soil is poisoned," he says. "It may just be that the pH is extremely low."

What you use to fix the balance of your soil depends on whether you want your garden to be 100 percent organic or not. True, "organic" gardening will restrict what you use for fertilization, as well as for pest control. (See "Resources" at the end of this chapter for suggestions on obtaining organic supplies.) For example, if the pH of your soil is too low, you can increase it by adding some limestone; if it's too high (above 7), you can decrease it by adding sulfur. A naturally mined mineral found in New Jersey called "green sand" will help soil with a low potassium level. The general concept of organic gardening, says Van-Vranken, "is creating a healthy soil so that you hopefully won't need any additional mechanisms to control pests."

Your garden should be at least two feet wide and as long as you desire. Most crops spread out at least two feet, so give them the space they need.

Seeds Versus Plants

Whether to plant seeds from scratch or start your garden with a little help from precultivated plantings basically comes down to convenience and cost. "When you plant several seeds, until you get some emerging, you don't know if they're going to amount to anything," VanVranken maintains.

Whereas several hundred lettuce seeds might cost $1, as compared to $4 or $5 for a six-pack of plants, out of those hundred seeds, very few will grow to "planthood." If you want your garden to look like a garden from the very beginning, you may want to consider just going with plants or seedlings. If you do, it's a good idea to also plant a few seeds as well, so your kids can observe and tend a flower or vegetable from its germination. Being "in charge" of a living thing from its earliest beginnings is a powerful feeling, even if you're only five.

One-Hundred Percent Organic?

Unless your chosen plants are certified "organic," they have likely been sprayed with a chemical pesticide. If you are going with seeds, look for ones that have not been genetically altered. If you're "container gardening," remember that the typical potting soil will normally have had nonorganic fertilizers added to it. You can buy organic potting soil, of which about a third will probably be composted manure.

FOOD FANTASY
Only Fanatics Eat "Natural" Foods

Once, not too long ago, when we thought of people who ate "natural" or "organic" foods, we envisioned food fanatics with long, unkempt hair, Birkenstock shoes, and ripped jeans. They not only wanted food that didn't destroy the earth in the process of being created, but they refused to eat things containing residues of toxic chemicals. Unless they grew their own food and spent hours in the kitchen, however, they didn't have a lot of choices. (Perhaps that's why they ate so much Grape-Nuts!)

But just as Birkenstocks have gone mainstream and jeans are now accepted at formal affairs, eating "natural" and "organic" is now associated with people of all ages and backgrounds who enjoy a healthy lifestyle. And organic convenience foods have likewise taken their places on supermarket shelves, letting you have your organic cake and eat it, too!

Caring About Compost

Basically, compost is the end result of organic material decomposing. By "organic," we don't mean in the sense of "organically grown," but as in things that were once living, such as plants, leaves, grass clippings, and vegetable peelings from the kitchen. Manure is another material that can be used in composting, but it must be handled in a safe manner, including making sure it's been "aged" at least 120 days. Compost is a natural way to add nutrients to your soil.

"Bacteria is the main organism that breaks the compost down," says VanVranken. But, he notes, "You're not looking for a sterile environment. What you are trying to do is to get the good bacteria to break it down into a form that allows it to crowd out the bad bacteria, which in many cases come from contaminated water or contaminated animal products" (one reason to avoid manure).

When composted properly—through the combination of heat (the inside of your compost pile will heat up to about 140 degrees Fahrenheit for a sort of "semipasteurization"), the presence of good bacteria, and adequate time—manure and other organic materials are safe to use. Manure products that have not been aged at least 120 days, VanVranken says, should not be used. Aside from causing dangerous bacteria problems, he cautions, if you were to put fresh manure under a plant, the massive release of ammonia likely to result would probably damage it.

You can locate your composting pile either in a bin or right on the ground. Composting, after all, is a natural process that is constantly going on. Take a walk in the woods and turn over some leaves. What you see underneath are other leaves that are composting. If, for appearance's sake, you would rather compost in a bin, you can make one out of almost any material—wood (but not the pressure-treated variety, which has had chemicals added to it), wire-mesh fencing, or concrete blocks. You can also buy a prefabricated composting bin. If you are building a bin, make it at least three feet by three feet. Construct only three sides; the bin should be open in the front and on top.

Five Steps to Compost

Making your own compost is not complicated and does not require a lot of space. Among its benefits is making better use of organic material such as vegetable scraps from the kitchen, leaves, and grass cuttings. Not only will you be recycling them, but you'll have less garbage to drag to the curb.

To make compost:

1. Start with an eight-inch layer of organic (once living) material, including kitchen scraps (such as fruit, potato, and vegetable peels), leaves, and grass cuttings. Do not use too

much grass, however, since grass depletes oxygen, delaying the composting rate. Do not add any meat scraps, grease, dog feces, or used cat litter. Water the organic material until fairly wet.

2. Add two inches of soil, which you can take directly from your garden. Water.
3. Add another eight inches of organic material. Water until fairly wet.
4. Add another two inches of soil. Water.
5. Repeat Steps 3 and 4 until the pile is about three feet high. This can be done all at one time or over a period of time.

When the contents of your compost bin or pile are about three feet high, you'll need to water and turn them (with a pitchfork) weekly. If you used any manure, make sure it "ages" for at least 120 days.

As an alternative to making a large compost pile (especially if you don't generate a lot of the material needed to build one), you can make a smaller one using a small prefabricated composting bin. The technique is still the same: Alternate layers of organic material with soil, keep the contents moist, and turn them weekly when the bin is full. Making compost is like steaming fresh spinach leaves: You end up with much less than you started with!

Ideally, you should have two compost bins—one that has completed the composting process and one that's in the works. Don't forget to add vegetable debris from your garden in the fall to your compost bin.

When your compost is ready to use (in about six to eight weeks, depending on what you're composting), it will be brown and crumbly, and will smell like the most wonderful soil after a spring rain. It can be added to your garden at any time, although some gardeners believe fall is best.

What Should I Grow?

Whether you're in an apartment or have several acres, the all-around easiest vegetables to grow are tomatoes. If you are container gardening, try the smaller varieties, which have minimal space requirements. After tomatoes, zucchini and summer squash are simple as well as abundant. Mini–summer squash versions are also available for small spaces.

Complex crops include sweet corn (a four- to twelve-foot-tall plant produces one ear), peas, and beans (which also require a lot of space for little return). Leafy greens such as lettuce and spinach are easy to grow, but they are cool-season crops, so need to be planted in the early spring.

What flowers you plant will depend on the location. Shade-loving plants such as impatiens will not thrive in full sun. Learn what your garden offers in terms of sun and shade, and you'll make better decisions once you get to the gardening store.

Whatever you grow, keep it off the ground. Plants that are droopy or fall over onto the soil stand a better chance of becoming infested with either a plant disease or unwanted insects. Use a trellis, stakes, or even barbecue sticks to prop them up.

"Bee" Kind to the Beneficials

Applying a chemical pesticide to your plants will not only expose your family to a toxic substance, but must be repeated; once is never enough. That's because pesticide use, like a drug habit, leads only to a need for more pesticides by either killing the beneficial natural predators of the target insects or sending them elsewhere in search of food. Bees, ladybugs, birds, lizards, frogs, and spiders are all friends of your garden. Invite them in (even put out a dish of water for them), treat them well, and you will receive much in return.

In your chemical-free garden, you will not only have more to do, but more to observe and to learn. As Aristotle said, "In all things of nature there is something of the marvelous." Unlike painting the house, you shouldn't regard tending your garden as a chore, but as a chance to interact with an unfolding, tiny piece of nature—and as a wonderful opportunity to involve your kids in the joys of doing so.

Now that you're more familiar with the benefits of buying organic, it makes sense to try and include as much organic food as possible in your grocery shopping (especially when purchasing ingredients for the recipes in the next chapter). Try to buy locally grown produce whenever possible. Best of all is anything that comes from your very own organic garden, which certainly will add to its appetite appeal!

RESOURCES

Organic Facts and News

The Organic Trade Association (OTA)
Web site: www.ota.com
Regulations, updates, and news about the organic industry, as well as organic information for the consumer.

Organic Gardening Supplies, Plants, Seeds, and Tips

Johnny's Select Seeds
Web site: www.johnnyseeds.com
Sells seeds and supplies, including fertilizer and organic plant food.

Mountain Valley Growers
Web site: www.mountainvalleygrowers.com
Sells certified organic herbs and perennials.

Natural Gardening Company
Web site: www.naturalgardening.com
   Sells organic flowers, herbs, and vegetable seedlings, as well as natural pest controls and fertilizers.

Organic Gardening Magazine
Web site: www.organicgardening.com
   Offers articles and tips related to organic gardening issues.

Seeds of Change
Web site: http://store.yahoo.com/seedsofchange/index.html
   Sells organic seeds and seedlings for vegetables, flowers, and herbs, as well as supplies, books, and gifts. Offers organic gardening advice and a monthly electronic newsletter. Also makes ready-made pasta sauce, grain dishes, and salsa, which are sold in many health-food stores.

Plant and Herb Information

Dr. Duke's Phytochemical and Ethnobotanical Databases
Web site: www.ars-grin.gov/duke/
   Searchable databases of plants using their common names. Also allow searching for plants with specific chemicals, for the activities of specific chemicals, and for plants or chemicals with specific activities.

8

Chemical-Free Cooking

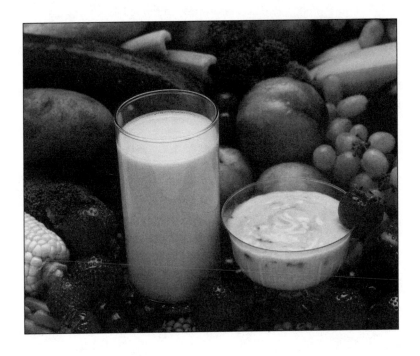

WHAT YOU'LL FIND IN THIS CHAPTER

How to make wholesome food as appealing to your kids as fast food. Smoothies and shakes can make breakfast a fun meal as well as a nutritious one, while salmon burgers are a great way to get your kids to eat fish that looks like "quarter pounders."

Not having enough time to cook doesn't mean you have to settle for additive-laden frozen fare. Great-tasting soups without the chemical ingredients found in the conventional varieties are a wonderful way to include a wide array of nutrients in your family's diet. Snacks and dips can also add to a healthy diet—provided they're the right kind. And wait until you try our winner dinner dishes!

Boot those sugary (or artificially sweetened) soft drinks from your fridge! They'll never be missed once your family has tasted the far better beverages you can easily whip together.

Food allergies and sensitivities need not condemn your family to the "bland blues." You'll be amazed at how the right recipes can do wonders for a restricted diet.

Did someone mention dessert? Here's how to end your meals on both a sweet and a nourishing note.

Cooking can—and should—be child's play. With the right preparation, even preschoolers can take an active role in preparing food.

Things You Can Do Right Now!

- Start cooking up a storm of healthy and delicious recipes.
- Serve them to your family, and they'll never want to go back to the "old way of eating."

So it all sounds great, but how do you go about making the transition from conventional to chemical-free cooking? Here are some recipes to help you bring your family the benefits of a healthier menu, including a special section for kids (and adults) who suffer from allergies or sensitivities to certain foods and ingredients.

Some of these recipes call for sugar. We hope you'll use organic sugar, such as turbanado or Sucanat (which is a brand name for an organic, less refined sugar with a high molasses content), instead of white, refined sugar. You can also use honey or molasses; however, when replacing a dry with a liquid sweetener, be sure to decrease the amount of liquid called for in the recipe. If you want to give cooking with stevia a try, you can use our conversion chart (see page 234), but don't expect baked goods to turn out exactly as they would with sugar. Whenever possible, use organic ingredients and whole-grain flours. It's becoming easier to purchase organic foods in your supermarket, but a well-stocked health-food store is still your best bet when it comes to finding organic ingredients.

ABOUT STEVIA

Some of our recipes call for stevia, which is a noncaloric, sweet-tasting herb sold as a dietary supplement in health-food stores. You will find concentrated stevia in liquid and powder form, although some of these products will have other ingredients to help preserve them or add bulk, since very little concentrated stevia is usually necessary.

Stevia has been used safely as both a flavoring agent and a sweetener for thousands of years in many countries. There have been no reports of any health-related complaints from the countless consumers who have used stevia, including diabetics. Nevertheless, the FDA has taken action against stevia distributors that the agency feels have implied that stevia is sweet (which it is) and can be used as a noncaloric replacement for sugar, aspartame, and other artificial sweeteners (which it can). This action, it should be noted, is not based on any reports of adverse effects, but rather appears to have been the result of a "trade complaint" made with the agency by an as-yet-unidentified company (reportedly an artificial sweetener manufacturer), which claimed stevia was an "untested" sweetener. So, because the FDA will not allow stevia to be categorized as a food additive, it can be purchased only as a dietary supplement and therefore does not include directions for use in cooking. (For more information on the FDA's actions against stevia, as well as safety studies and information on the herb, go to www.stevia.net or get a copy of *The Stevia Story* by Donna Gates and Linda and Bill Bonvie [B.E.D. Publications, 1996], or *The Miracle of Stevia* by James A. May [Twin Streams, 2003].)

If you're not familiar with stevia, the first thing to remember is that white, concentrated stevia is far sweeter than sugar and *cannot* be used as a cup-for-cup replacement for it. Too much stevia, in fact, will actually impart a bitter taste to foods. Not all the stevia products on the market taste the same; some have more of an aftertaste than others. Remember, stevia is a natural herb, not a laboratory creation, so there will always be differences in how any particular crop tastes depending on where it was grown and the type of stevia plant that was harvested. Some plants contain more of a certain type of glycoside that provides sweetness without any aftertaste.

You can also combine stevia and sugar, or stevia and honey, as a way to cut down on the sugar in a recipe or beverage.

If you want to replace the sugar in a recipe with stevia, or vice versa, see the conversion chart below.

STEVIA-SUGAR CONVERSION CHART

When cooking, if you want to replace the sugar in your recipe with stevia, use the following conversions as a guide.

Sugar	Stevia extract powder	Stevia extract liquid
1 cup	1 teaspoon	1 teaspoon
1 tablespoon	¼ teaspoon	7 to 9 drops
1 teaspoon	Pinch to 1/16 teaspoon	3 to 4 drops

Smooth Starters

Berry Smoothie

⤫

1½ cups almond or
  rice beverage
1 cup blueberries, fresh
  or frozen
1 cup strawberries, fresh
  or frozen

½ cup plain organic yogurt
2 to 3 tablespoons maple syrup,
  1 tablespoon honey, or a pinch
  of white stevia powder
1 tablespoon omega-3 and
  omega-6 oil blend* (optional)

Place all the ingredients in a blender and blend until smooth.
Pour into two glasses and serve immediately.

YIELD: 2 SERVINGS

*Udo's Choice, made by Flora, is a blend of flaxseed, evening primrose, and
omega-6 oils.

Chocolate Banana Smoothie

⤫

1 banana
1 to 1½ cups rice beverage or
  cow's milk (preferably organic)
1 tablespoon maple syrup

2 teaspoons organic chocolate
  powder (available in health-
  food stores)
3 to 4 ice cubes

Place all the ingredients in a blender and blend until smooth.
Pour into two glasses and serve immediately.

YIELD: 2 SERVINGS

Fruit Smoothie

1 banana
1 cup mixed fruit of your choice
⅔ cup fruit juice (not made
from concentrate or with
added sweeteners)

½ cup plain organic yogurt
2 tablespoons maple syrup
6 ice cubes

Place all the ingredients in a blender and blend until smooth. Pour into two glasses and serve immediately.

YIELD: 2 SERVINGS

Pineapple-Banana Breakfast Shake

½ cup pineapple juice
½ banana

½ cup plain yogurt or milk
(preferably organic)

Place all the ingredients in a blender and blend until smooth. Pour into two glasses and serve immediately.

YIELD: 2 SERVINGS

Recipe courtesy of the Feingold Association of the United States.

Kefir Smoothies

Breakfast Shake

∾

8 ounces plain kefir*
½ cup fresh or frozen fruit
1 to 2 tablespoons unsweetened,
   unsulfured coconut

½ to 1 teaspoon ground flaxseed
   or flaxseed oil
1 to 2 ice cubes (optional)

Place all the ingredients in a blender and blend until smooth.
Pour into two glasses and serve immediately.

YIELD: 2 SERVINGS

*We prefer Helios Nutrition kefir.

Sweet Kefir Smoothie

∾

8 ounces plain kefir*
½ cup fresh or frozen fruit of
   your choice
Natural flavorings such as
   cinnamon, nonalcoholic vanilla,
   or natural fruit flavorings,
   to taste

Pinch white stevia powder
   or 2 tablespoons honey

Place all the ingredients in a blender and blend until smooth.
Pour into two glasses and serve immediately.

YIELD: 2 SERVINGS

*We prefer Helios Nutrition kefir.

Other Breakfast Ideas

Basic Pancakes

∽

1 cup flour (preferably organic flour)
1 cup whole milk (preferably organic)
1 egg
¼ cup sugar

2 tablespoons oil
1 teaspoon baking powder
1 teaspoon pure vanilla
Dash salt

Preheat the grill or griddle.

Place all the ingredients in a medium-size bowl and mix well. Pour about ¼ cup batter onto the hot grill or griddle; cook until bubbles form and the edges are firm. Turn and brown the other side. Remove to a plate and cover to keep warm.

VARIATIONS: For whole-grain pancakes, substitute whole-grain flour for all or part of the flour. For cheese pancakes, add ½ to 1 cup shredded cheese to the batter. For nut pancakes, add ½ to 1 cup chopped nuts (except almonds) or seeds to the batter. (If you mix the batter in a blender, only the cook will know that nuts or seeds have been added. Peanuts work well and give a rich, wholesome flavor.)

YIELD: 12 (4-INCH) PANCAKES

Recipe courtesy of the Feingold Association of the United States.

Cheese Omelet

∽

2 eggs
2 tablespoons whole milk (preferably organic)

Salt (optional)
Butter
¼ cup grated or cubed cheese

In a cup or small bowl, beat the eggs, milk, and salt, with a fork. In a small frying pan over high heat, melt some butter. Pour in the egg mixture and stir slightly; cook until the mixture is no longer runny. Sprinkle in the cheese and carefully fold the omelet over itself.

VARIATIONS: Other fillings to use with or in place of the cheese include mushrooms, onions, avocado, bean sprouts, meat, or fish.

YIELD: 1 OMELET

Recipe courtesy of the Feingold Association of the United States.

Corn Cuties

1 cup brown rice flour
   baking mix *
1 to 2 cups fresh or frozen
   corn kernels
¾ cup milk or rice beverage

1 egg, slightly beaten
2 tablespoons coconut oil
½ teaspoon stevia liquid
   concentrate

Preheat the oven to 400 degrees. Lightly oil the cups of a minimuffin tin or line them with paper liners.

Place the baking mix in a large bowl and set aside. In a blender, combine the corn kernels, milk or rice beverage, egg, coconut oil, and stevia, and blend well. Pour the corn mixture into the bowl with the baking mix and stir until just blended; do not overmix. Spoon the batter into the prepared minimuffin tin, filling each cup approximately two-thirds full. Bake for about 12 minutes, or until a toothpick inserted in the center of a muffin comes out clean.

YIELD: 24 TO 36 MUFFINS

*Pamela's Products makes a delicious rice flour baking mix.

High-Fiber Oat-Bran Muffins

2½ cups oat bran (you can
   substitute oat flakes or rolled
   oats, but the muffins will have
   less fiber)
2½ cups grated raw sweet potato
   or 1¼ cups mashed banana
   plus 1¼ cups unsweetened,
   unsulfured coconut
1 tablespoon baking powder

1 teaspoon cinnamon
½ teaspoon salt
¼ teaspoon allspice
3 eggs, separated
1 cup water
2 tablespoons melted
   butter or coconut butter, or
   1 tablespoon of each

Preheat the oven to 400 degrees. Lightly oil the cups of a muffin tin or line them with paper liners.

In a large bowl, combine the oat bran with sweet potato or the banana and coconut. Add the baking powder, cinnamon, salt, and allspice, and mix well. Make a depression in the center of the mixture and add the egg yolks, water, and melted butter and/or coconut butter; mix well. In a separate bowl, beat the egg whites until slightly stiff and fold into batter. Spoon the batter into the prepared muffin tin, filling each cup about ⅔ full. Bake for 20 to 30 minutes, or until a toothpick inserted into the center of a muffin comes out clean. Let cool and serve with unsweetened organic apple butter, all-fruit jam, or very thin slices of peaches. Freeze any leftover muffins as soon as possible.

YIELD: 12 MUFFINS

Simple French Toast

1 egg   *1 slice whole-grain bread*
2 tablespoons milk or water

Preheat a griddle or pan to medium hot.
In a shallow dish, beat the egg. Add the milk or water, and combine. Dip the slice of bread in the mixture, coating both sides, and place in the griddle or pan. Fry until golden.

VARIATIONS: Add ¼ teaspoon vanilla to the egg mixture or sprinkle the fried bread with cinnamon.

YIELD: 1 SERVING

Recipe courtesy of the Feingold Association of the United States.

"For-Real" Fast Food

Cheese Crisp

1 whole-wheat or sprouted-   *Sliced black olives, sliced red*
   grain tortilla   *peppers, sliced mushrooms,*
Shredded cheddar and Monterey   *diced tomatoes, and/or*
   jack cheese   *diced jalapeño peppers, for*
                            toppings (optional)

Preheat the oven to 400 degrees.
Lay the tortilla out flat on a baking sheet and sprinkle with the shredded cheese all the way out to the edges. Dot with the toppings, if desired. Place the baking sheet on the center rack of the oven and bake until the cheese melts. Remove from the oven and allow to cool a bit, then slice into wedges with a pizza cutter and serve.

YIELD: 1 SERVING

Oven-Fried Chicken

୧୨

½ cup flour   ½ teaspoon salt
½ teaspoon onion powder   3 to 4 pounds chicken pieces

Preheat the oven to 425 degrees.

In a large plastic bag, mix together the flour, onion powder, and salt. Add the chicken pieces, two to three pieces at a time, and shake to coat. Arrange the coated chicken pieces in a large, shallow pan; do not crowd. Bake for about 50 minutes, or until done. Serve immediately.

VARIATIONS: Add additional seasonings such as ½ teaspoon thyme, ½ tablespoon dried parsley flakes, or ⅛ teaspoon pepper to the coating mix.

If you prefer to remove the chicken skin before cooking, lightly grease the pan and cover it during the first half hour of baking.

NOTE: Leftover pieces can be frozen individually and used for school lunches. Place a piece of frozen chicken in the lunch box in the morning; it will be thawed by lunch time.

YIELD: 24 TO 30 PIECES

Recipe courtesy of the Feingold Association of the United States.

Rice and Corn Burritos

୧୨

½ cup cooked organic basmati   1 whole-wheat or sprouted-
   or long-grain brown rice (this   grain tortilla*
   is a great way to use leftover   ⅓ cup salsa or to taste**
   rice from the day before)
¼ cup cooked fresh or
   frozen corn

Combine the rice and the corn in a steamer, and heat until warm. Warm the tortilla till soft and lay out flat. Spoon the rice and corn mixture down the middle of the tortilla; do not overfill. Top with the salsa to taste and roll up into a burrito. If desired, cut into halves or thirds, and serve.

YIELD: 1 TO 3 SERVINGS

*We prefer Food for Life organic sprouted grain tortillas.
**We prefer Seeds of Change organic medium picante salsa.

Salmon Burgers

∽

1 large can pink salmon   Onion flakes, to taste
2 eggs, slightly beaten   ¾ cup dehydrated potatoes*
Pepper, to taste

Preheat the oven to 350 degrees. Grease a large baking dish with olive oil.

Drain the salmon, saving the juice. Remove the bones and skin, and discard. Place the salmon in a large bowl and flake into small pieces. Add the eggs and pepper, and mix. Sprinkle with the onion flakes and add the dehydrated potatoes; mix well. If the mixture is too dry to form into patties, add some of the reserved salmon juice until mixture is moist enough to form patties. If the mixture is too wet, add more dehydrated potatoes. Form the mixture into hamburger-size patties and arrange in the prepared baking dish. Bake for 30 to 40 minutes, or until done. (The patties can be eaten either soft or crispy.) If desired, serve on whole-wheat buns and topped with organic ketchup, tomato slices, and baby greens.

YIELD: 6 LARGE OR 10 SMALL PATTIES

*We prefer Barbara's Brand instant mashed potatoes. Avoid supermarket brands, which usually contain preservatives.

WINNER DINNER DISHES

Alexander's Vegetarian Chili
∽

2 cans organic dark
   kidney beans
2 cans organic pinto beans
1 tablespoon chili powder

2 large cans organic
   whole tomatoes
1 tablespoon ground cumin

Place the beans in a large pot and mix. Add the chili powder. Place a strainer over the pot and pour in the tomatoes, letting the liquid drain into the pot; mix. Cut the tomatoes into bite-size pieces and add to the pot; stir well. Cook the mixture over low heat for about 30 minutes, or until hot. Serve with organic corn chips and sour cream, if desired. Store any leftover in the refrigerator for up to several days.

NOTE: If you wish to prepare a smaller amount, just halve all the ingredients.

YIELD: 8 TO 10 SERVINGS

Basic White Sauce

∽

2 tablespoons butter
2 tablespoons flour
¼ teaspoon salt (optional)

1 cup whole milk
(preferably organic)

STOVETOP: Melt the butter in a small saucepan over low heat. Blend in the flour and salt, stirring with a whisk until the mixture is smooth and bubbly; remove from the heat. Stir in the milk, return to the heat, and cook, stirring constantly, for about 1 minute, or until thickened.

MICROWAVE: In a small glass bowl, heat the butter in the microwave on medium for about 30 seconds, or until melted. Stir in the flour and salt. Gradually add the milk, stirring with a whisk until smooth. Heat for 5 minutes on medium, stirring occasionally.

VARIATIONS: To make cheese sauce, add ½ to ¾ cup (2 to 3 ounces) shredded cheese to the finished sauce and cook an additional minute.

Substitute chicken or turkey broth for the milk.

NOTE: Use this sauce in casseroles in place of condensed soup or add more milk, sliced mushrooms, sliced celery, and/or diced potatoes, and serve as a soup.

YIELD: 1 ½ CUPS

Recipe courtesy of the Feingold Association of the United States.

Chopped Chicken Salad

4 cups chopped cooked chicken
1 cup finely chopped red onion
1 cup finely chopped celery

1 cup finely chopped red
* bell pepper*
1 teaspoon sea salt

Vinaigrette

1 cup olive oil
½ cup apple cider vinegar
½ cup freshly squeezed
* lemon juice*
4 tablespoons Dijon-style
* mustard*

1 teaspoon freshly ground
* black pepper*
1 teaspoon dried rosemary
½ teaspoon sea salt
4 to 6 drops stevia liquid
* concentrate*

In a small bowl, whisk all the vinaigrette ingredients until well blended; set aside.

In a medium-size bowl, combine the chicken, onion, celery, bell pepper, and salt. Add the vinaigrette and toss until well mixed. Cover and refrigerate for several hours to allow the salad to marinate. Serve chilled over a bed of mixed field greens.

YIELD: 4 SERVINGS

Recipe courtesy of Donna Gates from *The Stevia Cookbook* (B.E.D. Publications, 1999).

Crock Pot Baked Beans

1 pound dry small white
* or navy beans*
¾ cup apple juice concentrate,
* thawed*
1 (6-ounce) can tomato paste
* or 1 ½ teaspoons paprika*
* (optional)*

1 tablespoon finely chopped
* fresh sweet basil or 1*
* teaspoon dried sweet basil*
1½ teaspoons salt
1 teaspoon dry mustard
* powder (optional)*
¼ teaspoon pepper

1 tablespoon finely chopped onion
  or 1 teaspoon dried onion
  flakes (optional)

To prepare the beans, the night before you plan to serve this dish, wash the beans by putting them in a strainer and rinsing them with cold water. Remove any shriveled beans. Put the beans in a 3-quart crock pot and fill the pot almost to the top with water. (The volume of the water should be two to three times the volume of the beans.) The next morning, pour the water off the beans and replace it with fresh water; repeat this two more times. (This soaking and rinsing process removes the indigestible carbohydrates that can cause gas.) Drain off all the water after the last rinse.

With the beans still in the crock pot, add 4 cups of water and put the lid on the crock pot. Cook the beans on high for 4 to 6 hours, or until very tender. Check the beans while cooking and add more water if necessary. It is okay for the water level to drop below the level of the beans.

In a small bowl, stir together the apple juice and tomato paste. Add to the crock pot along with the rest of the ingredients and stir well. Cover the crock pot and cook the beans on high for another 3 to 10 hours. Check the beans while cooking and add more water if necessary. Serve immediately, or refrigerate or freeze until needed.

For a thick sauce, smash some of the beans against the side of the crock pot about an hour before the end of the cooking time. If the sauce still isn't thick enough, set the lid ajar so that some of the liquid can evaporate. For very thick, oven-style baked beans, begin cooking the beans in the middle of the day. Add the seasonings and apple juice in the evening, and then cook the beans overnight.

YIELD: 8 TO 10 SERVINGS

Recipe used with permission from *Cooking 101: The Beginner's Guide to Healthy Cooking* by Nicolette M. Dumke (Allergy Adapt, 2002).

Easy Turkey over Toast

*½ pound turkey, cut into
  bite-size chunks ***
1 red pepper, diced
1 stalk celery, diced
*½ small red onion, finely
  chopped*

Salt and pepper, to taste
4 slices bread, toasted
4 sprigs parsley, for garnish

Sauce

*1 cup rice beverage or whole
  milk (preferably organic)*

½ cup shredded cheddar cheese
3 tablespoons organic flour

Prepare the sauce by heating the rice beverage or milk in the top
of a double boiler. When the liquid is heated, add the cheddar
cheese and stir. Add the flour slowly so that is doesn't form lumps
and stir well with a whisk.

When the sauce is well heated, add the turkey, red pepper, celery, onion, salt, and pepper; stir and cook until well heated.
Spoon over the toasted bread and garnish with the parsley.

YIELD: 3 TO 4 SERVINGS

*Use either leftover home-cooked turkey or a natural, no-additive, store-
made deli-counter turkey. The advantage of home-made turkey is that you
can buy organic poultry and be absolutely sure that nothing artificial has
been added. If you buy your turkey from a deli counter, have it cut in one big
chunk, not into sandwich-style slices.

Sweet and Sour Tempeh

⤜

2 (8-ounce) packages tempeh,
  cut into ½-inch cubes*
2 tablespoons olive oil,
  coconut oil, or butter
1½ large onions, diced
2 stalks celery, thinly sliced

1 large red bell pepper,
  coarsely diced
1½ cups water
1 teaspoon sea salt
4 cups cooked basmati rice

Marinade

½ cup tamari soy sauce
2 tablespoons apple cider
  vinegar
2 tablespoons water

4 cloves garlic, minced
⅛ teaspoon stevia liquid
  concentrate, or to taste

To prepare the marinade, combine the marinade ingredients in a small bowl or a 2-quart jar with a lid. If using a bowl, transfer the marinade to a gallon-size resealable plastic bag.

Add the tempeh to the marinade in the jar or bag, seal, and shake well to coat the tempeh. Allow the tempeh to marinate for at least 20 minutes and preferably for longer than an hour. (The longer the tempeh marinates, the tastier it will be.)

Heat the oil in a large skillet or a wok over medium heat. Add the onions and sauté for 3 to 4 minutes, or until translucent. Add the celery and bell pepper, and sauté for another 5 minutes, or until soft. Add the tempeh and marinade, and stir well; simmer, uncovered, for 10 minutes. Stir in the water and salt, cover, and reduce the heat to medium low; simmer for about 20 minutes. If desired, add additional stevia. Serve hot over the basmati rice.

YIELD: 4 SERVINGS

*We prefer Lightlife brand organic tempeh.

Recipe courtesy of Donna Gates from *The Stevia Cookbook* (B.E.D. Publications, 1999).

SENSATIONAL SOUPS

Soup can be a complete meal. Just add a salad, bread, and some fruit for dessert, and dinner is ready. Soups can cook nearly unattended while you do other things, so they fit well into a busy lifestyle. They also contain nutritious ingredients that are thoroughly cooked, so they are easily digested and the nutrients are well absorbed. Soups can be made almost effortlessly with a crock pot.

Chicken Broth

6 cups cold water
2 carrots, cut in half
2 stalks celery with leaves
1 to 2 onions, quartered
1 to 2 teaspoons chopped
    parsley

½ teaspoon garlic powder
10 peppercorns
Salt and pepper, to taste
2 to 3 pounds chicken breasts

In a deep kettle, combine all the ingredients except the chicken breasts. Heat slowly to the boiling point, then add the chicken, cover the kettle, and cook slowly until the meat is tender. Strain the broth and allow to cool. Refrigerate until the fat congeals then skim it off.

NOTE: You can freeze the broth in ice cube trays and then transfer it to containers for future use. The broth cubes thaw quickly, and you can take out just what you need.

YIELD: 6 TO 8 SERVINGS

Recipe courtesy of the Feingold Association of the United States.

Cream of Anything Soup

1 recipe Basic White Sauce   *2 cups water*
(see page 245)

Prepare the Basic White Sauce as directed. Add the water and heat until hot.

VARIATIONS: For cream of mushroom soup, chop ¼ to ½ pound fresh mushrooms and simmer in the 2 cups of water for about 10 minutes, or until tender. Add the water and cooked mushrooms to Basic White Sauce recipe as in the recipe above.

For cream of celery soup, substitute 2 to 3 cups of sliced celery for the mushrooms.

YIELD: 3 TO 5 SERVINGS

Recipe courtesy of the Feingold Association of the United States.

Down East Corn Chowder

3 cups fresh or frozen corn   *1 onion, finely chopped*
2 medium potatoes, peeled   *2 cups whole milk*
*   and finely chopped*   *   (preferably organic)*
2 cups Chicken Broth   *2 tablespoons butter*
*   (see page 250)*   *Salt and pepper to taste*

In a large pot, combine the corn, potatoes, Chicken Broth, and onion; cook until the potatoes and onion are tender. If desired, purée the mixture in a blender, then return to the pot. Add the milk and butter, and bring just to simmer. Add the salt and pepper, and serve hot.

YIELD: 4 TO 6 SERVINGS

Recipe courtesy of the Feingold Association of the United States.

Navy Bean Soup

∽

1 pound dry navy beans
3 stalks celery, sliced
2 carrots, peeled and sliced
3 tablespoons chopped fresh
  parsley or 1 tablespoon dry
  parsley
1 tablespoon chopped fresh
  sweet basil or 1 teaspoon
  dry sweet basil

2 teaspoons salt
½ teaspoon pepper (optional)
1 potato, peeled and grated
  (optional)

To prepare the beans, the night before you plan to serve this dish, wash the beans by putting them in a strainer and rinsing them with cold water. Remove any shriveled beans. Put the beans in a 3-quart crock pot and fill the pot almost to the top with water. (The volume of the water should be two to three times the volume of the beans.) The next morning, pour the water off the beans and replace it with fresh water; repeat this two more times. (This soaking and rinsing process removes the indigestible carbohydrates that can cause gas.) Drain off all the water after the last rinse.

With the beans still in the crock pot, add 6 cups of water along with the celery, carrots, parsley, sweet basil, salt, and pepper. Put the lid on the crock pot and cook the soup on high for 6 hours or on low for 8 to10 hours. Add the optional potatoes 2 hours before the end of the cooking time.

Check the soup near the end of the cooking time, and if it is thicker than you prefer, add some boiling water. Serve hot and freeze any leftover.

Yield: 2½ quarts

Recipe used with permission from *Cooking 101: The Beginner's Guide to Healthy Cooking* by Nicolette M. Dumke (Allergy Adapt, 2002).

Pat's Quick and Creamy Soup

⁓

2 cups Chicken Broth
(see page 250)
1 cup chopped broccoli or
other vegetable
2 tablespoons butter
½ small onion, chopped

¼ cup flour
1 cup milk (preferably organic)
Pinch pepper (white preferred)
Freshly grated parmesan
cheese, for garnish

In a medium-size saucepan, simmer the chicken broth and broccoli pieces for about 5 minutes, or until heated.

In a large saucepan, melt the butter over medium heat; add the onion and sauté until soft. Stir in the flour and brown slightly. Add the milk gradually, reduce the heat to low, and stir the mixture until well blended. Pour in the broth and broccoli, and stir. Heat, stirring, until the soup is thickened; do not boil. Add the pepper. Serve hot, sprinkled with the parmesan cheese.

YIELD: 3 SERVINGS

Recipe courtesy of the Feingold Association of the United States.

SMARTER SNACKS AND DIPS

Avocado Dressing
&

2 to 6 tablespoons water
1 small or ½ large avocado,
   peeled and pitted
2 tablespoons low-fat, live-
   culture yogurt or plain kefir

Juice of ½ lemon or lime
1 small garlic clove, crushed
Salt and freshly ground
   pepper to taste

Place 2 tablespoons of the water and the remaining ingredients in a blender or food processor and blend until smooth. If the mixture is too thick, add more water. Use immediately as a salad dressing or as a topping on baked potatoes garnished with vegetables such as chopped tomatoes, green onions, cucumber, and/or sweet red peppers. Refrigerate any leftover in a glass jar with a lid.

NOTE: Avocados are high in healthful fat. The avocado in this recipe is a substitute for other vegetable oils.

YIELD: ABOUT 1 CUP

Cool Kefir Dressing
&

2 cups fresh kefir*
1 heaping tablespoon chopped
   fresh parsley
1 heaping tablespoon minced
   fresh chives
1 heaping tablespoon finely
   chopped fresh lemon zest

1 heaping tablespoon finely
   chopped fresh garlic
1 teaspoon sea salt
¼ teaspoon Herbamare brand
   herbed sea salt
½ teaspoon xanthan gum

In a small bowl, combine all the ingredients except the xanthan gum; blend thoroughly. Slowly add the xanthan gum and continue to blend until the mixture thickens. Place in the refrigerator for 6 to 8 hours to allow the full flavor to develop.

Notes from Donna Gates: Dairy products combine best with nonstarchy vegetables and acidic fruits.
    Don't hesitate to add a little flaxseed oil to this recipe.

YIELD: 2 CUPS

*We prefer Helios Nutrition kefir.

Recipe courtesy of Donna Gates.

Cottage Cheese Dip

1 *cup low-fat cottage cheese*
¼ *cup plain low-fat yogurt,*
    sour cream, or mayonnaise
    (watch out for mayonnaise
    with "natural" flavorings)
½ *teaspoon salt*

¼ *teaspoon pepper*
3 *large radishes, finely chopped*
1 *carrot, grated*
2 *teaspoons caraway seeds*
    (optional)

Purée the cottage cheese with a hand blender, standard blender, or food processor until smooth. Add the yogurt, sour cream, or mayonnaise along with the salt and pepper, and purée again briefly. Stir in the radishes, carrot, and caraway seeds, and refrigerate until serving time. Serve with vegetable dippers such as broccoli florets, celery, and carrot sticks, or with healthy chips such as baked potato or corn chips.

YIELD: 1½ CUPS

Recipe used with permission from *Cooking 101: The Beginner's Guide to Healthy Cooking* by Nicolette M. Dumke (Allergy Adapt, 2002).

Fruit Balls

½ cup whipped cream cheese
1 teaspoon organic sugar
½ cup finely chopped organic
   prunes

½ cup finely chopped organic
   dates
Shredded unsweetened,
   unsulfured coconut

In a small bowl, combine cream cheese and sugar. Add prunes and dates, and mix well. Place the coconut in a separate bowl. Form the cream cheese mixture into small balls and roll the balls in the coconut.

YIELD: 16 TO 20 SMALL BALLS

Gorp

2 cups nuts and seeds of two
   or three different kinds (for
   example, peanuts and sunflower seeds; almonds and
   cashews; or pumpkin seeds,
   sunflower seeds, and almonds)

1½ cups raisins or other small
   or diced dried fruit
1 cup carob chips or grain-
   sweetened chocolate chips*

In a large bowl, mix all of the ingredients together. Put some in a plastic bag for your child to take to school for a healthy snack.

*An example is Sunshine brand chocolate chips, sweetened with malted barley and corn.

YIELD: 3½ CUPS

Recipe used with permission from Cooking 101: The Beginner's Guide to Healthy Cooking by Nicolette M. Dumke (Allergy Adapt, 2002).

Norma's Pear Sauce

cs͞o

6 pears, peeled, cored, and
    chopped
2 tablespoons water

2 tablespoons brown sugar
Dash ground cinnamon
Dash nutmeg

In a large saucepan, combine the pears and water; cover and cook over medium heat 20 minutes, or until soft. Add the brown sugar, cinnamon, and nutmeg, and stir until well blended. Serve hot or cold.

YIELD: 3 CUPS

Recipe courtesy of the Feingold Association of the United States.

DESSERTS

Baked Apples

cs͞o

6 tablespoons butter, softened
    to room temperature
Zest of 2 lemons
Juice of 2 lemons
¼ cup currants
¼ cup coarsely chopped
    almonds

½ teaspoon white stevia
    powder
1 teaspoon ground ginger
¼ teaspoon ground cloves
¼ teaspoon cardamom
6 large apples, quartered,
    peeled, and cored

Preheat the oven to 325 degrees. Lightly butter a baking pan.

In a large bowl, cream the butter with lemon zest and lemon juice. Add the currants, almonds, stevia, and spices, and stir. Place a spoonful of the mixture in each apple. Arrange the filled apple quarters in the prepared baking pan and add enough water to cover the bottom of the pan. Bake for 2 hours, or until tender.

YIELD: 6 SERVINGS

Recipe courtesy of Donna Gates.

Creamy Rice Pudding

∽

3 cups water
1 cup dry basmati rice
½ teaspoon sea salt
1 cup heavy cream
½ cup raisins
½ cup shredded unsweetened
  coconut

1 teaspoon cinnamon
½ teaspoon nutmeg
¼ teaspoon white stevia
  powder

Preheat the oven to 350 degrees.

In a 2-quart saucepan, bring 2 cups of the water to a boil over medium-high heat. Stir in the rice and sea salt, and bring to a second boil. Cover the pot, reduce the heat to low, and cook for 30 minutes, or until the rice is tender. Add the remaining water to the rice along with the remaining ingredients, and mix well. Spoon the mixture into an 8-inch casserole dish and sprinkle with additional cinnamon. Bake for 25 to 30 minutes, or until firm. Serve warm.

YIELD: 8 TO 10 SERVINGS

Recipe courtesy of Donna Gates.

Fruit Crisp

∽

Base

4 to 6 cups fresh fruit (good
  choices are blueberries,
  peaches, apples, and rhubarb)
¼ cup sugar (optional, if using
  tart fruit such as rhubarb)

1 tablespoon quick-cooking
  tapioca
½ teaspoon salt

Topping

1¼ cups rolled oats, uncooked   *¼ cup sugar*
¼ cup melted butter

Preheat the oven to 350 degrees. In a large bowl, combine the base ingredients; toss gently to mix. Let stand for 30 minutes, stirring occasionally. In another bowl, mix together the topping ingredients. Spread the base mixture in the bottom of an ungreased 9 x 9-inch baking dish, then cover it with the topping mixture. Place the baking dish in the oven and bake the dessert for 20 to 25 minutes, or until the top is lightly browned. Serve warm.

YIELD: 4 TO 6 SERVINGS

Lemon Pudding

4 cups peeled, coarsely diced   *3 cups water*
* yellow squash*   *4 heaping tablespoons agar flakes*
1 cup fresh lemon juice   * (available in health-food*
2 tablespoons finely chopped   * stores)*
* lemon rind*   *Sliced fruit, for garnish*

In a 2-quart saucepan, combine the squash, lemon juice, lemon rind, and 2 cups of the water. Cover and simmer over medium heat for about 10 minutes, or until the squash is soft. Purée by pushing through a fine sieve; set aside. In a small saucepan, combine the agar and the remaining water. Simmer over very low heat, stirring frequently, until the agar is completely dissolved. Add the squash mixture and simmer for another 5 minutes. Pour into a bowl and refrigerate for about 2 hours, or until gelled. Transfer to a blender and whip into a fluffy pudding. Spoon into serving dishes and refrigerate for another 30 minutes. Garnish with the fruit slices before serving.

YIELD: 6 (1-CUP) SERVINGS

BEVERAGES

Chocolate Syrup

∽

¼ *cup water*
½ *cup sugar*
¼ *cup cocoa*

¼ *teaspoon vanilla*
⅛ *teaspoon salt*

In a small saucepan, bring the water to a boil over high heat. Reduce the heat to medium and add the sugar and the cocoa; stir until dissolved. Remove the pan from the heat and stir in the vanilla and salt. Store in a glass jar with a lid and use by the teaspoon as a syrup for milk, ice cream, or other desserts. For each 8 ounces of milk, use about 2 to 3 tablespoons of syrup.

YIELD: ¾ CUP

Recipe courtesy of the Feingold Association of the United States.

Creamy Lime Delight

∽

1 *cup plain yogurt or kefir*
½ *cup freshly squeezed
    lime juice*

¼ *teaspoon stevia liquid
    concentrate or to taste*

Place all the ingredients in a blender and whip on high speed for 30 seconds. If the mixture is too thick, add some filtered water. Pour into two glasses and serve immediately.

YIELD: 2 SERVINGS

Recipe courtesy of Donna Gates from *The Stevia Cookbook* (B.E.D. Publications, 1999).

Frothy Pineapple Drink

1 cup water
1 cup whole milk (preferably
    organic)
1 (6-ounce) can frozen pine-
    apple juice concentrate

2 tablespoons sugar
1 teaspoon vanilla
6 to 8 ice cubes, crushed

Place all the ingredients in a blender and blend until smooth.
Pour into three or four glasses and serve immediately.

YIELD: 3 TO 4 SERVINGS

Recipe courtesy of the Feingold Association of the United States.

Hot Lemonade

6 to 8 ounces hot water
2 teaspoons lemon juice, or
    to taste

2 teaspoons honey, or to taste

Place all the ingredients in a large glass or mug, and mix well.
Serve immediately.

YIELD: 1 SERVING

Piña Colada Smoothie

⤲

1½ cups pineapple juice   1 teaspoon coconut flavoring
½ cup pineapple chunks   ⅛ teaspoon white stevia powder,
⅓ cup plain yogurt or kefir   or to taste

Place all the ingredients in a blender and whip on high speed for
30 seconds. Pour into two glasses and serve immediately.

YIELD: 2 SERVINGS

Recipe courtesy of Donna Gates from *The Stevia Cookbook* (B.E.D. Publications, 1999).

Watermelon Water

⤲

2 cups filtered or spring water,   ½ cup watermelon
   ice cold

Place all the ingredients in a blender and blend until frothy. Pour
into two glasses and serve ice cold for the best taste.

Note: Watermelon is an excellent source of lycopene, which is a very powerful antioxidant. Watermelon is also fat-free and a source of vitamins A, B_6,
C, and thiamin. On average, watermelon has about 40 percent more lycopene than raw tomatoes.

YIELD: 2 SERVINGS

COCONUT WATER KEFIR: A DAIRY-FREE
VARIATION OF A NATURAL HEALTH ELIXIR

Coconut water kefir is the invention of Donna Gates, a nutritional consultant and the author of the best-selling book *The
Body Ecology Diet*. A longtime advocate of kefir, Donna was

looking for a way to make the many benefits of kefir available to children and adults who cannot tolerate dairy, especially autistic kids who may be on diets free of milk protein. Donna's work with children who have been diagnosed with autism, ADD, or other learning disorders has shown that diet directly impacts the behavior of the children and the severity of their conditions. Many parents of such children who have incorporated coconut water kefir (as well as other dietary modifications and changes) have found an amazing difference in the way their kids function. Donna's work has led her to believe in the critical nature of what's known as the "gut-brain connection." She firmly believes that correcting problems in the gut and restoring a healthy "inner ecosystem" can benefit every system in the body.

Coconut water kefir is made from the water of young green coconuts. It is a mineral-rich elixir that Donna also claims has wonderful cleansing properties, aids in digestion, increases vitality, and even stops the craving for sugar.

To make coconut water kefir, you'll need Body Ecology's kefir starter culture (see "Resources" at the end of this chapter), at least three young coconuts, and a clean, airtight, glass container.

The young green coconuts you find in Asian markets and health-food stores usually aren't green. When they're sent to the United States, the green husk is cut off, so what you see is a white husklike covering. To get to the liquid, use a sharp object such as a screwdriver or corkscrew to make a hole in the center, then just pour out the water.

Make sure that the water from the coconuts is not cold. If you've been storing the young coconuts in the refrigerator, you'll need to heat the water a little bit, to about 92 degrees Fahrenheit (skin temperature), before you add the starter. If the water is too cold, it won't ferment.

Once the water has been warmed, pour it into the glass jar and mix in the kefir starter culture. Screw on the jar lid and let the jar sit at room temperature for at least twenty-four hours. The longer the kefir is allowed to ferment, the more sour it will be. If it's winter and your kitchen is cold, the fermentation may take much longer, so you may want to place the jar in a Styrofoam container or insulated lunch box, or even wrap it in a towel and stow it in the pantry. The ideal temperature for kefir to ferment is 70 to 72 degrees Fahrenheit.

When the kefir is done, its color will change to a milky white. Often, it will have a bit of a "skin" and bubbles on top. When you open the jar, you'll hear a little "whooshing" sound, which indicates that beneficial organisms have been growing in there. Another way to tell if kefir is done fermenting is to taste it. It should taste tart and tangy, a sign that all the sugar is gone. If, after twenty-four hours, your kefir doesn't appear to have finished fermenting, you can close up the jar and let it continue fermenting. When the kefir is "done," transfer it to the refrigerator for storage.

To make a new batch of kefir (which you can do as least seven times from one starter packet), you should retain anywhere from a few tablespoons to two inches of your current batch in the jar and add the water of three new young coconuts; seal up the jar and start the process all over again. The more of your old batch you use, the more sour the new batch will be. The kefir you use to start your new batch should be taken out of the refrigerator about an hour before you're ready to use it. In addition, slightly warm the water from the new coconuts so that your new batch will be about 92 degrees when you add the starter culture.

Because coconut water kefir doesn't have much of a taste (it's a little sparkly, tingly, and sour), it can be flavored very easily using other liquids and flavorings such as unsweetened cranberry juice and stevia. Donna recommends that both adults and children drink about four ounces of kefir four times a day (for a daily total of about sixteen ounces). She suggests having some at breakfast, at midday, and at bedtime. Some of the autistic children with whom Donna works drink up to two big glasses a day. "What we're doing with the autistic kids is mixing about four ounces of coconut water kefir and a couple ounces of black currant or cranberry juice with a little stevia to sweeten it," says Donna. She adds that adults often like it mixed with sparkling mineral water.

To learn more about coconut water kefir and other cultured foods, go to Donna's Body Ecology Web site (see "Resources" at the end of this chapter). You may also want to check out the Body Ecology bulletin board found at the Web site for a forum related to children, diet, and learning disabilities.

ALLERGY AND SENSITIVITY SPECIALS

While cooking for picky eaters may test your patience, having a kid with food allergies or sensitivities may make you feel as if your only job is being a chef. Nicolette M. Dumke, author of *Cooking 101: The Beginner's Guide to Healthy Cooking* (Allergy Adapt, 2002) and *5 Years Without Food: The Food Allergy Survival Guide* (Allergy Adapt, 1998), has developed recipes that answer the question of "what is left to eat" when faced with food allergies. As she says regarding the difficulty involved in being on a special diet, "How can we live and cope with food allergies, and in the process achieve good health? Three things are necessary: the right diet, a practical means of implementing the diet and staying on it, and most important of all, the right attitude."

The following delicious recipes will please everyone in your house, even those not on a restricted diet. More information about food allergies can be found at Nicolette Dumke's Web site at www.food-allergy.org.

Banana Sorbet
❧

2 bananas
2 to 3 tablespoons Fruit Sweet*
    or honey to taste (optional)

Cut the bananas into chunks, put the chunks into a plastic bag,
and place the bag in the freezer for several hours or overnight.
(Banana chunks can be frozen for an extended period of time.)

When ready to prepare the sorbet, remove the chunks from
the freezer and let them stand at room temperature for 10 minutes. Purée them with a hand blender, standard blender, or food
processor until smooth. (If using a hand blender, process the chunks
in two batches using the cup that came with the blender.) If desired, blend in the sweetener. Serve immediately as a smooth, creamy
dessert, freezing any leftover. Remove the leftover from the freezer
about 20 minutes before serving.

YIELD: 2 TO 4 SERVINGS

*Fruit Sweet is a peach, pear, and pineapple juice concentrate made by Wax
Orchards.

Recipe used with permission from *Cooking 101: The Beginner's Guide to
Healthy Cooking* by Nicolette M. Dumke (Allergy Adapt, 2002).

Gingerbread
❧

2 cups whole-wheat or 2³⁄₈ cups   ¾ teaspoon ginger
    whole-spelt flour*   ½ cup molasses
2 teaspoons baking powder   ½ cup water
1 teaspoon cinnamon   ¼ cup oil

Preheat the oven to 350 degrees. Oil and flour an 8- or 9-inch
square cake pan.

In a large bowl, stir together the flour, baking powder, and spices. In a separate bowl or cup, combine the molasses, water, and oil. Stir the liquid ingredients into the dry ingredients until just combined. Pour the batter into the prepared pan; bake for 30 to 40 minutes, or until browned and a toothpick inserted into the center of the cake comes out dry. Remove from the oven and cool on a wire rack.

YIELD: 1 CAKE

*We prefer Purity Foods whole-spelt flour.

Recipe used with permission from *Cooking 101: The Beginner's Guide to Healthy Cooking* by Nicolette M. Dumke (Allergy Adapt, 2002).

Kamut Shortbread Cookies

2½ cups kamut flour
½ teaspoon baking soda
½ cup plus 2 tablespoons apple
  or pineapple juice concentrate,
  thawed

½ cup oil

Preheat the oven to 350 degrees.

In a large bowl, stir together the flour and baking soda. In a separate bowl or cup, combine the juice and oil; mix well. Stir the liquid ingredients into the dry ingredients to form a stiff dough. Turn the dough out onto a baking sheet and roll to about a ¼-inch thickness with a rolling pin. Using a sharp knife, cut the dough into 2-inch by 3- to 3½-inch rectangles. Bake for 20 to 25 minutes. Remove the baking sheet from the oven and cut the cookies on the same lines again. Remove the cookies from the baking sheet with a spatula and put them on paper toweling to cool completely.

YIELD: 2 TO 3 DOZEN COOKIES

Recipe used with permission from *5 Years Without Food: The Food Allergy Survival Guide* by Nicolette M. Dumke (Allergy Adapt, 1997).

Lentil-Barley Soup

∽

1⅓ cups dry lentils
2 stalks celery, sliced
2 carrots, sliced
½ cup pearled barley
1 (14-ounce) can diced
 tomatoes

1 teaspoon salt
¾ teaspoon dried sweet basil or
 2 teaspoons chopped fresh
 sweet basil
¼ teaspoon pepper

To prepare the lentils, the night before you plan to make this soup, wash the lentils by putting them in a strainer and rinsing them with cold water. Remove any shriveled or bad-looking lentils. Put the lentils in a large saucepan and fill the pan almost to the top with water. (The volume of the water should be two to three times the volume of the beans.) The next morning, pour the water off the lentils and replace it with fresh water; repeat this two more times. (This soaking and rinsing process removes the indigestible carbohydrates that can cause gas.) Drain off all the water after the last rinse.

With the beans still in the saucepan, add 8 cups of water along with the celery, carrots, and barley. Bring to a boil over medium to medium-high heat, then reduce the heat and simmer for 1 hour. Check the soup occasionally and add additional water if necessary.

At the end of the hour, add the tomatoes, salt, sweet basil, and pepper, as well as 1 to 2 additional cups of water if needed. Simmer for another 15 to 30 minutes. Remove from the heat and serve hot.

YIELD: 4 TO 6 SERVINGS

Recipe used with permission from *Cooking 101: The Beginner's Guide to Healthy Cooking* by Nicolette M. Dumke (Allergy Adapt, 2002).

Pineapple Sorbet

᭟

20-ounce can pineapple chunks or
tidbits packed in their own juice

Place the can of pineapple in the freezer for several hours or overnight. (Pineapple chunks and tidbits can be frozen for an extended period of time.)

When ready to prepare the sorbet, remove the can of pineapple from the freezer and let it stand at room temperature for 10 to 20 minutes. Open the can on both ends and push the pineapple chunks out. Purée the chunks with a hand blender, standard blender, or food processor until smooth. (If using a hand blender, process the pineapple in two batches using the cup that came with the blender.) Serve immediately as a smooth, creamy dessert, freezing any leftovers. Remove the leftovers from the freezer about 20 minutes before serving.

YIELD: 2 TO 4 SERVINGS

Recipe used with permission from *Cooking 101: The Beginner's Guide to Healthy Cooking* by Nicolette M. Dumke (Allergy Adapt, 2002).

Spelt Muffins

2½ cups whole-spelt flour
3 teaspoons baking powder
¼ teaspoon salt (optional)
1 cup apple juice concentrate,
thawed
⅓ cup oil

Optional additional ingredient
(choose one): 1 cup fresh or
solidly frozen blueberries; ⅔ cup
peeled and diced apple or pear;
⅔ cup diced dried fruit such as
apricots, dates, apples, peaches,
or papaya; ⅔ cups raisins;
⅔ cup chopped nuts; ⅓ cup nuts
plus ⅓ cup diced dried fruit or
raisins; or 2 tablespoons lemon
or orange peel (just the outer
colored zest)

Preheat the oven to 350 degrees. Lightly oil the cups of a muffin tin or line them with paper liners.

In a large bowl, mix together the flour, baking powder, and salt. In a separate bowl or cup, combine the apple juice and oil. Add the liquid ingredients into the dry ingredients and stir until just mixed. Gently fold in the optional additional ingredient. Spoon the batter into the prepared muffin tin, filling each cup about ⅔ full. Bake for 20 to 25 minutes. Remove the muffins from the cups and place on a wire rack to cool.

YIELD: 11 TO 14 MUFFINS

Recipe used with permission from *Cooking 101: The Beginner's Guide to Healthy Cooking* by Nicolette M. Dumke (Allergy Adapt, 2002).

Spice Cake with Date Frosting

3 cups barley flour
¾ cups date sugar
3¾ teaspoons baking powder
½ teaspoon salt
2 teaspoons cinnamon
½ teaspoon cloves

¼ teaspoon allspice
3 cups puréed or thoroughly
  mashed bananas
½ cup plus 1 tablespoon oil
1 teaspoon vanilla extract
  (optional)

Date Frosting

⅔ cup water
1½ tablespoons barley flour

1 cup date sugar

Preheat the oven to 375 degrees. Oil and flour an 8- or 9-inch square cake pan. (Flour the pan with barley flour to make a completely wheat-free cake.)

To prepare the cake, in a large bowl, stir together the 3 cups barley flour, ¾ cups date sugar, baking powder, salt, and spices. In a separate bowl, combine the mashed or puréed bananas, oil, and vanilla. Stir the banana mixture into the flour mixture until just combined. Pour the batter into the prepared pan (the batter will be thick), and bake for 45 to 50 minutes, or until browned and a toothpick inserted into the center of the cake comes out dry. Remove from the oven and cool on a wire rack.

Meanwhile, to prepare the frosting, combine the water and 1½ tablespoons barley flour in a small saucepan. Heat the mixture over medium heat, stirring frequently, until it thickens and boils. Add the 1 cup date sugar and stir until smooth. Remove from the heat and use immediately to frost the top of the spice cake. Allow the cake to cool, then cut it into squares and serve it from the cake pan.

YIELD: 1 FROSTED CAKE

Recipe used with permission from *Cooking 101: The Beginner's Guide to Healthy Cooking* by Nicolette M. Dumke (Allergy Adapt, 2002).

COOKING CAN—AND SHOULD—BE
CHILD'S PLAY

If Mollie Katzen had her way, all kitchens would come equipped with kid-geared food-preparation zones, including tables just right for preschoolers to work at, long wooden spoons for stirring, serrated (not *sharp*) dinner knives with colored plastic tape on the handles to remember where your hand goes, an electric skillet, and lots of paper towels and sponges.

Katzen, host of *Mollie Katzen's Cooking Show* on public television and author of the legendary *Moosewood Cookbook* (Ten Speed Press, 1972) as well as *Pretend Soup* (Tricycle Press, 1994) and *Honest Pretzels* (Tricycle Press, 1999), believes children— very young children—can and should cook. Not as your helper, but as head chef, with you as the stand-by assistant. It's a bit of a role reversal, but Katzen knows from experience that kids are up to the challenge. Not only does food preparation give them a sense of accomplishment and enjoyment (not possible when meals appear from the mysterious kitchen and are put in front of them), but also motivates them to actually *eat* foods that they wouldn't even have looked at before.

Pretend Soup, a cookbook for kids as young as preschool age, accomplishes just that. With recipes in two versions—one for grown-ups that includes safety tips and food preparation chores best left to an adult and one for kids with the steps shown in pictures—the book gets kids involved in cooking. Katzen believes that once you get kids involved in some phase of meal preparation, be it planning, selecting, or cooking, you've crossed a major hurdle in getting them to eat a healthier diet.

Tips from Mollie

- Don't serve just plain veggies—make them taste good! Use salt, butter, shredded cheese, and toppings that will encourage even picky eaters.

- Take your kids with you to a farmers' market to buy vegetables. There will be no distractions like those that produce whining in the supermarket, such as candy and cookie aisles. Let them take part in the selection, or better yet, have them pick a recipe, make a list, and then find the items themselves.
- Never leave a child alone when cooking.
- Try to do everything on a child's level.
- Don't let the child put things in the oven or take them out; only adults should do these steps.
- Don't worry about the mess. "Have a sense of humor . . . spills are what sponges are for!"
- A child should *never* use a sharp knife, only serrated dinner knives and strong plastic ones.
- Let the child select what to make as often as possible.
- Always set things up properly before starting to cook.
- As the adult supervisor, always be watchful and aware of what's going on in the kitchen.

RESOURCES

Chemical Sensitivity and Environmentally Friendly Products

NEEDS, Inc.
Post Office Box 580
East Syracuse, NY 13057
Telephone: 800-634-1380
Web site: www.needs.com

Offers chemical sensitivity and environmentally friendly products including health and beauty aids, household items such as cleaning supplies, nutritional supplements, books, and air and water purifiers. Products are available online and by mail order.

Organic and Natural Food Sources

Annie's Naturals
792 Foster Hill Road
North Calais, VT 05650
Telephone: 802-456-8866 or 800-434-1234
E-mail: sarah@anniesnaturals.com
Web site: www.anniesnaturals.com
   Offers natural salad dressings, condiments, and marinades, including several organic salad dressings. Products are available online and in supermarkets and health-food stores.

Barbara's Bakery
3900 Cypress Drive
Petaluma, CA 94954
Telephone: 707-765-2273
E-mail: info@barbarasbakery.com
Web site: www.barbarasbakery.com
   Offers cereals, crackers, cookies, chips, and snack bars made without preservatives, artificial ingredients, hydrogenated oils, or refined white sugar. Products are available in supermarkets and health-food stores.

Eden Foods
701 Tecumseh Road
Clinton, MI 49236
Telephone: 888-441-3336
E-mail: info@edenfoods.com
Web site: www.edenfoods.com
   Offers organic beans, chips, condiments, soy beverages, fruits and juices, oils, pastas, barley malt syrup, tomato and sauerkraut products, and vinegar. Products are available online and in health-food stores.

The Grain and Salt Society
273 Fairway Drive
Asheville, NC 28805

Telephone: 800-TOP-SALT (867-7258)
Fax: 828-299-1640
E-mail: topsalt@aol.com
Web site: www.celtic-seasalt.com
Offers a wide variety of food products, teas, seasonings, and kitchen accessories, with a focus on Celtic sea salt. Products are available online and by telephone.

Helios Nutrition Kefir
214 Main Street
Sauk Centre, MN 56378
Telephone: 888-3 HELIOS (343-5467)
Fax: 320-351-8500
E-mail: helios@heliosnutrition.com
Web site: www.heliosnutrition.com
Offers organic, ready-to-drink dairy kefir. Products are available in health-food stores.

Horizon Organic
6311 Horizon Lane
Longmont, CO 80503
Consumer Hotline: 888-494-3020
Web site: www.horizonorganic.com
The nation's first and leading producer of certified organic dairy products. Offers juices, milk, yogurt, cheese, butter, and eggs. Products are available in supermarkets and health-food stores.

Kashi
Post Office Box 8557
La Jolla, CA 92038
Telephone: 858-274-8870
Web site: www.kashi.com
Offers natural, minimally processed cereals, bars, shakes, and mixed-grain instant cereal for infants. Products are available online and in supermarkets and health-food stores.

Lundberg Family Farms
5370 Church Street
Post Office Box 369
Richvale, CA 95974-0369
Telephone 530-882-4551
Fax: 530-882-4500
E-mail: question@lundberg.com
Web site: www.lundberg.com
Offers organic brown rice, specialty rice varieties, and brown rice products. Products are available online and in supermarkets and health-food stores.

Odwalla
120 Stone Pine Road
Half Moon Bay, CA 94019
Telephone: 650-726-1888
Email: consumer@odwalla.com
www.odwalla.com
Offers natural, "flash pasteurized" juices (including several organic flavors), smoothies, shakes, spring water, and a variety of fruit, grain, and nut bars. Products are available online and in select supermarkets and health-food stores.

Organic Valley Family of Farms
CROPP Cooperative
507 West Main Street
LaFarge, WI 54639
Telephone: 888-444-6455
E-mail: organic@organicvalley.com
Web site: www.organicvalley.com
The largest organic farmer–owned cooperative in North America, with more than 460 farmer members in seventeen states. Offers milk, butter, cheese, eggs, juice, and meat. Products are available in supermarkets and health-food stores.

Pamela's Products
335 Allerton Avenue

South San Francisco, CA 94080
Telephone: 650-952-4546
Fax: 650-742-6643
E-mail: info@pamelasproducts.com
Web site: www.pamelasproducts.com
Offers wheat- and gluten-free cookies, biscotti, and baking mixes. Products are available in health-food stores.

Rice Dream
1245 San Carlos Avenue
San Carlos, CA 94070
Telephone: 650-595-6300
E-mail: questions@imaginefoods.com
Web site: www.imaginefoods.com
Offers a nondairy rice beverage made from organic or premium California brown rice in original flavor, vanilla, and chocolate, with or without added calcium and vitamins A and D. Products are available in supermarkets and health-food stores.

Seeds of Change
Post Office Box 15700
Santa Fe, NM 87506
Telephone: 888-762-7333
E-mail: gardener@seedsofchange.com
Web site: www.seedsofchange.com
Offers 100 percent organic pasta sauces, salad dressings, salsas, frozen entrées, rice, and grains, as well as organic seeds, seedlings, and garden supplies. Products are available online.

Small Planet Foods
719 Metcalf Street
Sedro-Woolley, WA 98284
Telephone: 800-624-4123
Web site: www.cfarm.com
One of the country's leading producers of organic food products under the Cascadian Farm and Muir Glen labels. Offers

frozen fruits and entrées, canned tomatoes, salsas, and pasta sauces. Products are available in supermarkets and health-food stores.

Spectrum Naturals
1304 South Point Boulevard
Suite 280
Petaluma, CA 94954
Telephone: 707-778-8900
Fax: 707-765-8470
E-mail: Info@SpectrumOrganic.com
Web site: www.spectrumorganic.com
   Offers unrefined, organic, and semirefined vegetable oils, condiments such as canola mayonnaise, a nonhydrogenated margarine, organic low-fat and fat-free salad dressings, and organic vinegar. Products are available in supermarkets and health-food stores.

Stonyfield Farm
Ten Burton Drive
Londonderry, NH 03053
Telephone: 800-776-2697
Web site: www.stonyfield.com
   Offers organic and nonorganic yogurt (including whole milk yogurt packaged for kids) in a variety of flavors, organic cultured soy, organic premium ice cream, and organic frozen yogurt. Products are sold online and in supermarkets and health-food stores.

U.S. Mills
200 Reservoir Street
Needham, MA 02494-3146
Telephone: 781-444-0440
Fax: 781-444-3411
Web site: www.usmillsinc.com
   Offers Erewhon brand organic cereals and New Morning brand organic cereals and graham crackers. Products are available in health-food stores.

Westbrae Natural
The Hain Celestial Group
734 Franklin Avenue
Suite 444
Garden City, NY 11530
Telephone: 800-434-4246
Web site: www.westbrae.com
    Offers vegetarian beans, soups, pastas, vegetables, condiments, Japanese products, and rice and soy beverages. Products are available in health-food stores.

White Wave/Silk
Web site: www.whitewave.com
    Offers organic soy products such as soy beverages, tempeh, and tofu under the White Wave and Silk labels. Products are available in supermarkets and health-food stores.

Organic and Natural Food Stores

Diamond Organics
Post Office Box 2159
Freedom, CA 95019
Telephone: 888-ORGANIC (674-2642)
E-mail: info@diamondorganics.com
Web site: www.diamondorganics.com
    A complete organic grocery store (and more) online, with guaranteed overnight delivery in the United States. Available items range from produce and dairy products to organic cotton clothing for infants to wine and bread.

Whole Foods
601 North Lamar
Suite 300
Austin, TX 78703
Telephone: 512-477-4455

E mail: rs.team@wholefoods.com
Web site: www.wholefoods.com
The world's largest retailer of natural and organic foods, with 139 stores across the United States.

Wild Oats
3375 Mitchell Lane
Boulder, CO 80301
Telephone: 800-494-9453
E-mail: info@wildoats.com
Web site: www.wildoats.com
A nationwide chain of natural and organic food markets, with ninety-nine stores in twenty-three states and Canada. The stores include Wild Oats Natural Marketplace, Capers Community Markets, Henry's Marketplace, and Sun Harvest.

Organic and Natural Pet Foods

Epetfood.com
Spectrum Pet Foods, Inc.
1000 Lewis Street
Montgomery City, MO 63361
Telephone: 800-354-2832
E-mail: spectrum@ktis.net
Web site: www.epetfood.com
Offers organic food for dogs, cats, kittens, birds, small animals, reptiles, and fish, as well as hypoallergenic and special-needs dog and cat foods. Products are available online and at select pet food stores and veterinarian offices.

The Honest Kitchen
1804 Garnet Avenue
Suite 201
San Diego, CA 92109
Telephone: 858-483-5995
E-mail: info@thehonestkitchen.com
Web site: www.honestkitchen.com

Offers 100 percent, human-grade dog food containing organic ingredients, as well as a food for dogs that are intolerant to grains and a canine nutritional supplement. Products are available online.

Organic Baby Food and Products

Earth's Best
Web site: www.earthsbest.com
Offers a full line of ready-made organic baby foods including cereals, beginner foods, juices, teething biscuits, whole-grain bars, cookies, and apple sauce, all with no added salt or sugar. Products are available online and in supermarkets and health-food stores.

Organic Bébé
233 Harvard Boulevard
Lynn Haven, FL 32444
Telephone: 866-734-2634 or 850-271-4345
E-mail: mail@organicbebe.com
Web site: www.organicbebe.com/products.asp
Offers natural skin and hair care products, cloth diapers, organic clothing, bedding, and baby food. Products are available online.

Tender Harvest
Web site: www.tenderharvest.com
Offers a complete line of organic baby foods from Gerber. Products are available in supermarkets and health-food stores.

Stevia and Kefir Products

Body Ecology
273 Fairway Drive
Asheville, NC 28805
Telephone: 800-511-2660
Fax: 770-234-5453

E-mail (for product information): orders@bodyecologydiet.com
Web site: www.bodyecologydiet.com
    Offers stevia products as well as a kefir starter kit to make co-
conut water kefir. Products are available online and in health-
food stores.

The Herbal Advantage
131 Bobwhite Road
Rogersville, MO 65742
Telephone: 417-753-4000
Fax: 417-753-2000
E-mail: info@herbaladvantage.com
Web site: www.herbaladvantage.com
    Offers a full line of stevia products. Products are available on-
line and by mail order.

Stevita Company
7650 US Highway 287
Suite 100
Arlington, TX 76001
Telephone: 888-783-8482 or 817-483-0044
Fax: 817-478-8891
E-mail (for product information): mail@stevitastevia.com
Web site: www.stevitastevia.com
    Offers a full line of stevia products. Products are available by
mail order and in health-food stores.

Wisdom Herbs
2546 West Birchwood Avenue
Suite 104
Mesa, AZ 85202
Telephone: 800-899-9908
E-mail: wisdom@wisdomherbs.com
Web site: www.buywisdomherbs.com
    Offers a full line of stevia products. Products are available on-
line and in health-food stores.

Afterword

The process of removing toxic influences from your home, your environment, and your family's diet is one that can unfold piece by piece. But be assured that each change will make a difference, no matter how insignificant it may seem at first.

We hope that after reading this book, you'll think about things from a different perspective. The blind faith that we, as consumers, have afforded commercial interests has been grossly misplaced. We have been lied to, cheated, and deceived. We have been told over the years that cigarettes are good for digestion, that fluoride is a necessary nutrient, that leaded gasoline is a "gift from God." We have seen artificial colorings, food additives, and pesticides continue to be blithely consumed and accepted by the public as "safe," even as more and more of them are deemed too hazardous by regulators to go on being marketed.

Frequently, studies will hit the news with both soothing and confusing headlines, classifying something we suspected of being dangerous as being safe, and vice versa. We're exposed to so much conflicting information that we tend to become desensitized to warnings and cautions about everything from toxic pesticides to artery-clogging trans fats. But that, after all, is the job of public relations experts: to spin information in a way that puts us at ease about the products we use and keeps us in the dark about the real issues—and about the toxic threats to our children's health and well-being.

Childhood represents a window of opportunity for bringing out hidden potentials, but also a window of vulnerability to often hidden dangers. Not only are children more susceptible to the toxic effects of chemicals and food additives, but steering them clear of such substances at an impressionable age might very well direct the choices they make as adults. We are the role models for our kids, the most important people in their lives, at least for a short time. By introducing them to a chemical-free lifestyle—if only a step at a time—and allowing them to become active participants in the process, we are helping to imbue them with habits that hopefully will result in their living longer, healthier, happier, and more productive lives.

Notes

CHAPTER 1

1. Russell Blaylock, *Excitotoxins: The Taste That Kills* (Albuquerque, NM: Health Press, 1996), page 71.
2. "Children's Special Vulnerability to Environmental Risks," *Natural Resources Defense Council*, www.nrdc.org/default.asp.
3. Ibid.
4. Ibid.
5. Interview with Dr. Philip Landrigan, February 2001.
6. Ibid.
7. Robert S. Mendelsohn, *How to Raise a Healthy Child . . . In Spite of Your Doctor* (New York: Ballantine Books, 1987), page 104.
8. "GAO Releases Report on Study of Pesticide Use in Schools," *U.S. Environmental Protection Agency*, www.epa.gov/iaq, February 2002.
9. Carol Simontacchi, *The Crazy Makers: How the Food Industry Is Destroying Our Brains and Harming Our Children* (New York: Putnam, 2000), page 186.
10. "Trans Fatty Acids: A Hidden Killer," in "On Health," *Web MD*, http://webmd.com, June 5, 2000.
11. Peter Montague, "Some Dangers of Hormones in Milk," *Rachel's Hazardous Waste News* #382, http://www.ejnet.org/rachel/rhwn382.htm, March 24, 1994.
12. European Union Scientific Committee on Veterinary Measures Relating to Public Health, "Report on Public Health Aspects of the Use of Bovine Somatotrophin," March 15–16, 1999.
13. *Pure Facts: Newsletter of the Feingold Association of the United States*, June 2000.
14. Eric Schlosser, *Fast Food Nation* (New York: Houghton Mifflin, 2001), pages 263–264.
15. "Our Children at Risk," *Natural Resources Defense Council*, www.nrdc.org/default.asp.

16. Interview with Dr. David Wallinga.
17. Interview with Adam Goldberg.
18. Interview with Dr. Philip Landrigan.
19. Simontacchi, page 84.
20. Simontacchi, pages 185–186.

CHAPTER 2

1. Feingold Association of the United States, *Diet, Learning & Behavior* (booklet).
2. *Neurobehavioral Toxicology*, volume 1, pages 41–47.
3. Jane Hersey, *Why Can't My Child Behave?* (Alexandria, VA: Pear Tree Press, 1996), pages 68–69.
4. J. Kowalchuk, "Antiviral Activity of Fruit Extracts, *Journal of Food Science*, volume 41 (1976), pages 1013–1017.
5. Hersey, page 66.
6. Hersey, page 67.
7. Feingold Association.
8. Eric Schlosser, *Fast Food Nation* (New York: Houghton Mifflin, 2001), pages 126–127.
9. Ruth Winter, *A Consumer's Dictionary of Food Additives,* Fifth Edition (New York: Three Rivers Press, 1999), page 391.
10. James S. Turner, "Foreword," in Donna Gates and Linda and Bill Bonvie, *The Stevia Story* (Atlanta, GA: B.E.D. Publications, 1996).
11. Russell Blaylock, *Excitotoxins: The Taste That Kills* (Albuquerque, NM: Health Press, 1996), pages 35–36.
12. Ibid., pages 42–47.
13. Ibid., page 66.
14. Ibid.
15. Blaylock, page 80.
16. Blaylock, page 74.
17. Linda and Bill Bonvie, "The Cane Mutiny," *New Age Journal*, April 1999.
18. Jean Carper, *Food: Your Miracle Medicine* (New York: Harper-Collins, 1993), page 303.
19. James S. Turner, "The Aspartame/NutraSweet Fiasco," www.stevia.net/aspartame.htm, 2000.
20. Blaylock, page 39.
21. Simontacchi, pages 187–188.

22. Ibid., pages 185–186.
23. Blaylock, pages 211–213.
24. Feingold Association, pages 1–2.

CHAPTER 3

1. "Marketing Food and Drinks to Kids," *Reuters Business Insight*, http://www.reutersbusinessinsight.com/default.asp.
2. Ibid.
3. Donna Gates, *The Magic of Kefir* (Atlanta, GA: B.E.D. Publications, 1996), page 18.
4. "Marketing Food and Drinks to Kids."
5. Allan Magaziner, *The Complete Idiot's Guide to Living Longer and Healthier* (New York: Macmillan Distribution, 1998).

CHAPTER 4

1. U.S. Environmental Protection Agency, Office of Pesticide Programs, "Chlorpyrifos Revised Risk Assessment and Risk Mitigation Measures," www.epa.gov/pesticides/op/chlorpyrifos/consumerqs.htm.
2. Cornell University Program on Breast Cancer and Environmental Risk Factors in New York State, "Chlorpyrifos Fact Sheet."
3. Mount Sinai School of Medicine, Center for Children's Health and the Environment, "Chlorpyrifos Fact Sheet."
4. "What Is a Pesticide?" *Journal of Pesticide Reform*, Summer 1999.
5. Michael Hansen, *Escape from the Pesticide Treadmill: Alternatives to Pesticides in Developing Countries* (N.p.: International Organization of Consumers Unions and Pesticide Action Network, 1988).
6. Ibid., page 14.
7. Ibid., page 16.
8. Ibid., page 22.
9. U.S. Environmental Protection Agency estimate, 1999.
10. "Our Food, Our Future," *Organic Gardening*, September–October 2000.
11. "Study Focuses on Weed-Killer in Water," in "Food & Health," *CNN.com*, August 17, 1995.
12. Interview with Antonio Bravo, U.S. Environmental Protection Agency.
13. Interview with Daniel Swartz.

14. Interview with Richard Wiles.

CHAPTER 5

1. Yamhil County (Oregon) Solid Waste Division.
2. "Indoor Air Quality Page," *U.S. Environmental Protection Agency*, www.epa.gov/iaq.
3. *Rachel's Environment and Health Weekly*, volume 250.
4. Ibid.
5. Arnold Mann, "When Mold Takes Hold," *USA Weekend*, July 19–21, 2002.
6. Diana Crumpler, *Chemical Crisis* (Carlton, Australia: Scribe Publications, 1994), pages 10–11.
7. Linda and Bill Bonvie, "Something in the Air," *New Age Journal*, August 1994.
8. Ibid.

CHAPTER 6

1. Bruce P. Lanphear et al., "Cognitive Deficits Associated with Blood Lead Concentrations Below 10 mg/dL," *Public Health Reports*, http://phr.oupjournals.org, March 2001.
2. U.S. Environmental Protection Agency, Technology Transfer Network, National Air Toxics Assessment, Lead Compounds, www.epa.gov/ttn/atw/nata/conf.html.
3. Ibid.
4. Ibid.
5. "Poisonous Pastime," *Violence Policy Center*, www.vpc.org/studies/leadintr.htm, May 2001.
6. "Proposed Rules: Metal-Cored Candle Wicks Containing Lead and Candles with Such Wicks: Notice of Proposed Rulemaking," *Federal Register*, volume 67, number 79, April 24, 2002.
7. "Lead Content of Calcium Supplements," *Journal of the American Medical Association Women's Health*, volume 284 (September 20, 2001), pages 1425–1429.
8. Ibid.
9. *The Human Brain Protection: History's Lead Story*, The Franklin Institute, http://sln.fi.edu.

10. "History of Precaution," part 2, *Rachel's Environment and Health Weekly*, volume 540.

11. National Safety Council, Environmental Health Center, Lead Testing Information.

12. Ibid.

13. "Health Care Without Harm," Center for Health, Environment and Justice, www.noharm.org.

14. Rep. Dan Burton, "Autism: Present Challenges, Future Needs: Why the Increased Rates?" opening statement, Government Reform Committee, U.S. House of Representatives, April 6, 2000.

CHAPTER 7

1. Cheryl Long, senior editor, *Organic Gardening*. Letter to then–Secretary of Agriculture Dan Glickman.

2. *British Food Journal*, volume 99, number 6 (1997), pages 207–211.

3. Cheryl Long.

4. Rod MacRae, *Strategies for Overcoming the Barriers to the Transition to Sustainable Agriculture*, Ph.D. thesis, McGill University, 1990.

5. Rodale Institute, brochure, 1999.

6. Conella H. Meadows, "Our Food, Our Future," *Organic Gardening*, September-October 2000.

7. Interview with Jeff Moyer.

8. B. P. Baker, C. M. Benbrook, E. Groth III, and K. L. Benbrook, "Pesticide Residues in Conventional, Integrated Pest Management (IPM)—Grown and Organic Foods: Insights from Three U.S. Data Sets," *Food Additives and Contaminants*, volume 19, number 5, (May 2002) pages 427–446.

9. *Journal of Pesticide Reform*, volume 19, number 2 (Fall 1999), pages 2–7.

PERMISSIONS

The photo on page 3 is used courtesy of the U.S. Department of Agriculture/ARS Photo.

The fish consumption advice on pages 33–34 is used courtesy of the Environmental Working Group (www.ewg.org).

The photo on page 37 is used courtesy of the U.S. Department of Agriculture/Ken Hammond.

The photo on page 69 is used courtesy of the U.S. Census Bureau.

The information in Table 3.1 on page 83 is from *Food: Your Miracle Medicine* by Jean Carper, copyright © 1993 HarperCollins. It is used courtesy of HarperCollins.

The photo on page 105 is used courtesy of the U.S. Department of Agriculture/Doug Wilson.

The photo on page 133 is used courtesy of the U.S. Department of Agriculture/Ken Hammond.

The information in Table 5.1 on pages 136–139 is used courtesy of Enviroene, a part of the Environmental Protection Agency Web site (http://es.epa.gov).

The Intelligent Pest Management Tips on pages 156–158 were adapted from *The Bug Stops Here: How to Safely and Simply Control Most Household Pests Without Harming Yourself or Your Family* by Steve Tvedten, copyright © 1998, 1999, 2000, 2001, 2002 by Steve Tvedten. It is used with permission from Steve Tvedten.

The photo on page 173 is used courtesy of the U.S. Department of Agriculture/Ken Hammond.

The information in "Are You Planning to Buy or Rent a Home Built Before 1978?" on page 180 is used courtesy of the U.S. Environmental Protection Agency.

The tips to protect against lead exposure on pages 186–188 are used courtesy of the U.S. Environmental Protection Agency.

The instructions for cleaning up the mercury after a thermometer breaks on pages 197–198 are courtesy of the Center for Health, Environment and Justice, Falls Church, Virginia.

The photo on page 211 is used courtesy of the U.S. Department of Agriculture/ARS Photo.

The photo on page 231 is used courtesy of the U.S. Department of Agriculture/ARS Photo.

Index